For Warren & Virginia,
God's Blessings!

Praise for Roxanne
Struck Down *but* NOT Destroyed

Roxanne Smith is an amazing person! Lying horizontal up to 22 hours a day because of chronic pain, she still lives a full and fulfilling life—wife, mother, friend, Stephen Minister, author. Roxanne doesn't gloss over her challenges nor deny her pain, tears, and limitations. But her faith, hope, and joy in Christ are vibrant and inspiring.

Rev. Kenneth C. Haugk, Ph.D.
Founder and Executive Director of Stephen Ministries
St. Louis, Missouri (www.stephenministries.org)
Author of *Journeying through Grief* and
Don't Sing Songs to Heavy Heart.

Roxanne's story of triumph in the midst of great difficulty is a testimony to her spirit, her perseverance, and her zest for life. This is a story meant to inspire others. Roxanne and Andy, have built a team of supporters, committed to promoting the health of body, mind, and spirit. Roxanne has been the leader of this team. I am grateful for my opportunity to be a part of Roxanne's health promotion team, and a witness to her heroic life.

Dr. Mitchell Elkiss
Osteopathy, Neurology, Acupuncture
Farmington Hills, MI

Roxanne Smith has been there. If you have had your life turned upside down in the course of moments, hours, or weeks, Roxanne knows your grief, your despair, your helplessness. If you're nowhere close to the life you expected and hoped for, the life that seemed the natural 'next step,' Roxanne knows what you're experiencing.

With insight and maturity born of tribulation and spiritual wrestling, Roxanne invites you to journey with her and her traveling companions... Roxanne offers help in understanding what the journey can mean and how God can bless your life in the midst of—or because of—your pain.

Ruth N. Koch, M.A., NCC
Social Worker, Counselor
Speaker, Author
Denver, CO

Roxanne traces her days – always defined by pain – as a mother, a wife, a friend, and now an author. Extensive detail regarding each exploration of hope seemed unnecessary... but how like someone who is pain free to want to move along even when reading – because details slow life down. The author wisely forces the reader to slow down and experience her life.

Grace Hughey
Community Life Director
St. John Lutheran Church
Ellisville, MO

Struck by disabling pain so severe, Roxanne's life has been forever altered in ways that oppose her basic nature. Her faith, fortitude and resilience are a testimony to what a person can endure when they take one problem at a time...You will find a coach, a friend and a resolve that can help you gain your victory.

Stephen Hower
Senior Pastor
St. John Lutheran Church
Author of *Sharpening the Sword*
and other titles

Roxanne shares the conversation between her and dear friends who are part of a support group, unique heart-felt poetry, her psychiatrist's perspective on illness, and even a letter from her son. These personal gems make the book truly unique and open one's heart up to hear her message... Her unwavering cheerful attitude shows her true faith more than any healing could ever provide.

Lisa Copen
Rest Ministries, Director
HopeKeepers Magazine, Editor
National Invisible Chronic
Illness Awareness Week
Founder & Coordinator

STRUCK DOWN
but NOT
*D*estroyed

Finding *Hope* in the Maze of Suffering
By Roxanne M. Smith

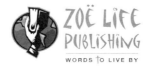
ZOË LIFE
PUBLISHING
WORDS TO LIVE BY

Published by:
Zoë Life Publishing
P.O. Box 871066
Canton, MI 48187 USA
www.zoelifepub.com

Author: Roxanne M. Smith
Cover Designer: Chamira Jones
Editorial Team: Sabrina Adams, Pamela Gossiaux and Jessica Colvin

First U.S. Edition 2008 Softcover, Perfect Bound

Summary: A young, newly married bride finds herself in a sudden onslaught of back pain--severe enough to cause her to lie down all but two hours a day, at best! This is a story of perseverance through her painful way of life as she seeks God's help to have a child, have a wonderful marriage, and be the strong successful woman she was meant to be.

10 Digit ISBN 1-934363-18-9 Soft Cover
13 Digit ISBN 978-1-934363-17-1 Soft Cover

Library of Congress Control Number: 2008933927

For current information about releases by Roxanne M. Smith or other releases from Zoë Life Publishing, visit our website: http://www.zoelifepub.com

Printed in the United States of America

v7.6 09 14 09

Thanks and Acknowledgments

To Kathie Supiano, for kindly but persistently urging me to write about my journey with pain.

To B.J. Connor, my close writer friend, for the experience and wisdom she shared.

To Lloyd Stuhr, for first suggesting that my suffering might help others.

To Pastor David Koch, for his excellent advice on editing this manuscript.

To Ruth Koch, for her encouragement and inspiration.

To our small group: Sean, Lisa, Allen, Sandi, Shannon, Carla, Jim, Krissa, and Andy—for sharing their stories and for encouraging me to tell mine.

To the group of proofreaders, Carla, Laura, Betty, Wendy, Pam K., Pam P., Steve, Sharon, Barb, Ernie, Judy, Pete, Anne, Jan, Julie, Cindy, Marilee, and Gertrude, thanks for all your comments in the margins and for suggesting missing subchapters.

To Pastor Ted and Becky Jungkuntz—for being my cheerleaders and helping me craft a title.

To Pastor and Arline Zehnder, for their love and affirmation.

To Andy, my intimate companion on this journey, thank you for the countless hours spent word processing to help me make changes in the manuscript. Thank you for helping me to interpret these many experiences so that I could capture them in words. I love you.

To Jakob, for helping me to believe that I could be a good mom despite my disability. Thank you for wanting other disabled adults to consider parenting.

To Sabrina Adams, for answering God's call to start a publishing house—Zoë Life—and for being my substantive editor.

To Sherry Perkins, who first made me aware of Zoë Life.

To Pam Gossiaux, my very qualified copy editor.

To Chamira Jones, for her creative cover design and artistic layout.

To Jessica Colvin, for helping me around the final bend.

To my parents, whose unflagging support has been a tremendous asset of stability in my life for many years. Thanks, Mom and Dad!

To the Stephen Ministers at St. Luke Lutheran Church, for their prayer support and conviction that this book could be used in Christian care giving.

To the St. Luke Women's Ministry, Special Needs Ministry, MOPS group, and Youth Group, for inviting me to speak about my experiences, and to practice telling my story.

To my friends at Community Bible Study in Ann Arbor. Thanks for setting up my cot each week so I could join you!

To all those doctors and health care professionals who treat patients with kindness and compassion, who truly see them as fellow human beings, and who try to help as possible.

STRUCK DOWN
but NOT
*D*estroyed

Finding *Hope* in the Maze of Suffering
By Roxanne M. Smith

Table of Contents

Preface

This is the book I wish I could have read eighteen years ago when life as I knew it suddenly and traumatically fell apart. During my first twenty-seven years, I had the world by the tail—successful student, athlete, musician, physical therapist, and engaged to a great guy. I was reduced from being a jock—biker, hiker, skier, you name it—to an invalid "horizontal woman" who has to lie down most of the time to manage excruciating back pain.

Degenerative disc pain stole my career and my "normalcy." What do you do when prayers for healing seem to fall on deaf ears? When "the problem of pain" isn't theoretical but a daily, throbbing reality that affects every aspect of your life?

I felt like I had been struck down and couldn't get back up. I felt like I was trapped in a maze and couldn't find my way out. We tried almost everything to relieve my pain and return me to a normal life. I desperately wanted to get out of the maze of suffering. But God kept leading me down another turn in the maze.

I hoped to be healed and THEN write about what I learned. Since complete physical healing hasn't occurred, I'm writing this anyway. I describe how my faith in God sustains me through continued suffering. It is possible to live victoriously in the midst of suffering. And everyone faces some type of suffering. I'm writing to give others hope.

So, dear reader, I hope this speaks to you, from my heart and life experience to yours. My prayer is that you gain enough strength or courage to keep going for another day, or that you can encourage someone you love to hang in there for another day.

Introduction

I am a horizontal woman.[1] I must spend twenty-two of every twenty-four hours lying down. I eat meals lying down. I travel in our van lying down. The few times during the day when I'm standing up are counted in minutes, not hours. It isn't weak leg muscles, or undeveloped bones, which have made me this way; rather, it's pain. You see, I spent the first twenty-seven years of my life as a vertical woman, living a normal lifestyle. Just the last eighteen have been horizontal. Severe back pain from degenerative disc disease has forced this radical change into my life.

Pain is my burden, but function is my currency. The two hours or so per day when I can be vertical are my most carefully-rationed resource. They are more valuable to me than money. How will I spend my two hours? Every day I have to budget that time, as if it were a short stack of ten dollar bills. Each time I do something while standing up, I have to hand one of the bills in. I do things quickly, because the clock is ticking. A shower is a priority: brushing my teeth can't be ignored. There's fifteen minutes gone already. Exercise needs to be next: driving myself to the pool, changing, carefully swimming a few laps, stretching, changing, driving myself home again. That takes about one-and-a-half hours. So now I have about fifteen minutes left. Walk to the mailbox; fold a few items of clothing; empty the dishwasher. Time's up!

Now I can eke a little more time out of my back by being half-way between vertical and horizontal: semi-reclined. I can check my e-mail from a reclining chair and write a message or

---

[1] Berger, Suzanne E., Horizontal Woman: The Story of a Body in Exile, Houghton Mifflin Company, 1996.

two. I can lean forward over a single step and do some scrap-booking on the floor or write a card to a friend or even prepare a few vegetables for cooking. From then on, the rest of my day is lying down. For the rest of the day, I have a date with my daybed, like it or not.

On days I don't go swimming, I might use twenty minutes to take a walk. Once a week, I volunteer at a school for half an hour, helping with reading. Or, I might do some light shopping for thirty minutes to an hour. And that's it—that is the sum of my vertical life. There's no sitting at all, to speak of—unless it's ten minutes or less.

I am physically able to be vertical for longer than two hours each day, but, oh, at what a price. The times I've tried standing or sitting longer have caused excruciating pain flares which go on for weeks, if not months. When that happens, I have to go back on full bed rest for days until my tissue calms down enough to allow a few minutes of function again. Then come several weeks of gradually increasing activity, trying to regain "my normal" two hours of rationed function. Pain flares become a game of survival and test my coping ability to the max.

So, having learned my limits the hard way, I go on living my carefully managed life. "How have you coped?" you may ask. "What do you do with your time each day?" "Can't modern medicine help your condition?" "Or, if not correct it, can't modern medicine at least give you pharmaceutical pain relief?"

This book is my attempt to answer these questions. But it's about more than just answering questions. It's about overcoming life challenges. It's about playing the cards you are dealt, especially when you think you've been dealt a bad hand! It's about discovering that you can still have meaning and purpose in your life even if you don't get the "happy ending." It's about being content but not satisfied...being in a situation, praying for healing or for something to change... but while praying and waiting, also maximizing the moment which God has given.

I've learned many things in eighteen years which might be helpful for others who live with pain. I write this book by hand, lying down on my daybed in the living room. My terrific husband Andy bought me an anti-gravity pen[2] so I can write with the pen tip pointed either sideways or upward and not run out of ink. Andy has patiently typed the text into my laptop computer, line by line, as I've read it to him out loud. He has willingly and painstakingly entered my revisions. On good days I've done a little word-processing myself. This writing project, like all projects and goals which I set for myself, must be adapted to my horizontal life.

To understand my story, I have to take you back in time, so you can see where I've been and how trauma and recovery fit into my life. Please allow me to show you a quick view of my vertical years before I describe the horizontal life I now lead.

---

[2] originally designed for astronauts in the space program!

CHAPTER ONE

My Vertical Life

Growing Up Able-Bodied in Iowa

I was born in Iowa and grew up there, the fourth of five children: three girls and two boys. My father was a pastor and my mother a homemaker who was busy taking care of her growing family. Although we lived in a city, both of my parents were raised in the country and grew up in the Midwest during the Great Depression. During this difficult time between the two world wars they learned to be hard working, self-reliant, and resourceful. They learned how to face hard times with courage and hope. As their children we were taught those values and many practical life skills. My sisters and I learned to sew, bake bread, cook, grow a garden, can and freeze its produce, and—for fun—play the piano. My brothers learned woodworking, handyman skills, gardening, and how to play the piano.

My parents also passed down a strong faith tradition and belief in God, born out of a German Lutheran heritage. Our ancestors emigrated from Germany in the mid-1800s. We attended church regularly and spent time reading the Bible at home, but it was more than just religion. My parents emphasized having a lifelong relationship with God. They taught us how to walk through life seeing all things through the lens of faith in Him.

The German work ethic we inherited was an asset in school, and our parents encouraged us to do our best in whatever we set out to do. Both of our parents had college educations and our dad had the equivalent of a master's degree as well, so both emphasized reading and the value of education. As a result, three out of five of us were high school valedictorians, and one a salutatorian. We all have college degrees and three of us have either Master's degrees or other graduate work. We were also taught patriotism and our older brother served in the Vietnam War.

Arriving at the end of this large family, my brother Pete and I were very close in age but quite a bit younger than our siblings. We spent most of our time playing together in an age before computers, video games, cable TV, DVD players and the Internet, so we were very active. Our free time was spent riding bikes, climbing trees, walking on stilts, and hanging out at the swimming pool for hours. It seemed like we were always in motion. Winters brought incredible opportunities for sledding, snowball fights, building forts, and making snowmen. We didn't stop with snow people but added snow dinosaurs which we colored by pouring pitchers of green water over the frozen snow.

To my mother's chagrin I became a tomboy. She would

try to clean me up in the cute little dresses she sewed for me, sometimes with a matching coat or hat, and I'd tolerate that just so long before I'd throw on a pair of shorts under my dress and go hang upside down on the monkey bars! We have a great picture of me at age five playing with a bucket of mud, my doll face-down in the dirt next to my bucket.

Pete and I also created plenty of mischief. We were fascinated by the way that grass clippings in water gradually turned brown and smelly if you put them in a plastic container together. Our poor mother warned us not to do that, but the science experiment was *irresistible!* We were punished when she found a number of old margarine tubs hidden in window wells around the house. It was worth it — seeing something rot was so *awesome!*

In fifth grade I began to play the clarinet in school, and by seventh grade my band director asked me to also start playing the oboe. I enjoyed marching band, concert band, and orchestra. My brother Pete played the trombone, and with all the piano players in our home it was a musical place. Sports-wise, I started playing basketball, took tennis lessons, and learned how to golf.

By high school I had been put into accelerated math and science, so I was able to take Physics, Chemistry, and Calculus before graduating. Because of my strengths in these areas I was advised by my high school counselor to consider majoring in engineering.

I began college in Biomedical Engineering at the University of Iowa. After one year I changed my major to pre-physical therapy because I liked the idea of working directly with patients. My time at the university was not particularly happy, however; the academic competition was intense, as the

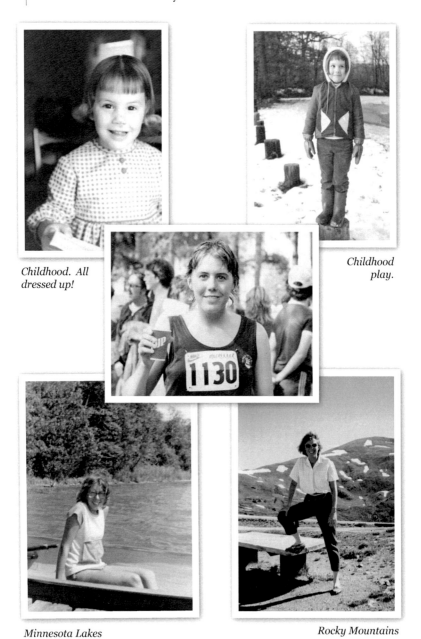

Childhood. All dressed up!

Childhood play.

Minnesota Lakes

Rocky Mountains

Middle center: After running a 10k race.

large lecture classes of several hundred were filled with pre-med and pre-dental school students. I put in many long hours studying. It was a lonely and often sad time for me. During this time, I suffered with an eating disorder, which I later learned had been a "maladaptive (unhealthy) coping mechanism" for my loneliness.

I studied during my junior year at Concordia University in Seward, Nebraska, where my brother Pete was also in college. The campus was small and friendly and I was much less lonely. This was a more intimate school that allowed me to know my science professors personally. Along with five other students, I took advantage of an interim course with Prof. Joe Gubanyi, to travel to Florida for three weeks. We camped in the Everglades, snorkeled on the coral reefs, and backpacked through much of the natural areas of the state. It was a wonderful, hands-on learning experience. For my senior year, I returned to the University of Iowa, since at that time, Concordia did not have a pre-physical-therapy option.

In spite of the eating disorder, I continued to work hard, and I graduated *summa cum laude*. During this time, I gradually gained recovery from the eating disorder. I was helped by going through a twelve-step program similar to Alcoholics Anonymous, but for food addictions. After graduation I went on to University of Iowa's program in physical therapy. This wonderful program involved two years of graduate work, including dissecting a cadaver in anatomy class and doing three internships. I made some great friends and really enjoyed these years. After passing the board exam, I received my physical therapy license and moved to southeast Michigan for my first job. My oldest sister, Barb, lived in Ann

Arbor, and I wanted to live near her.

What a great time that was! I was finally done with school, studying, and exams. I loved my job working with patients at McPherson Hospital in the small town of Howell. There was finally some money to spend during free time because my job paid a good salary. It seemed like an ideal time to have fun, so a friend and I joined a bike riding group and we often rode thirty miles on Saturday mornings. Other friends that I met through my job loved cross-country skiing. We did that together, sometimes going away for the weekend to the "snow belt" of Michigan midway up the state. One weekend we cross-country skied twenty-six kilometers!

My apartment complex had walking trails which I used for running, and it had tennis courts which I enjoyed as well. I felt a sense of freedom and happiness doing athletic activities, especially outdoors and with good friends, which was unmatched by anything else in life. I loved adventure. My apartment mate, Karen Eischer, enjoyed camping near Lake Michigan, so we did that several times. We had a saying that there wasn't anything in life that three days on Lake Michigan couldn't cure!

An opportunity arose to work in outpatient orthopedics so I changed jobs and eventually moved into sports medicine. There, I treated patients and supervised an athletic trainer. We specialized in treating knee, ankle, and shoulder injuries in patients much like myself: young, active, and healthy. It was a wonderful, busy, active time for me. I really couldn't imagine life being any other way.

Dating, Engagement, Pain Breaks In!

In 1988, I began dating two different young men at about the same time. Both Andy and Matt* went to my church, and both were teachers. Each asked me out in September, even though I didn't know either one of them very well. I enjoyed going out to dinner or dancing and decided it might be fun to get to know each of them—it certainly would allow me to compare the two, and decide if either were compatible with me. My apartment mate and good friend, Karen Eischer, knew both Andy and Matt. She thought it was a grand experiment, and she helped me sort out my thoughts and feelings after going on a date.

Andy took me to an Oktoberfest, a German dinner and dance with a polka band. I found him to be friendly, intelligent, and an excellent conversationalist. We had a good time, talking for several hours. He was reluctant to dance, though, and in general didn't seem very athletic.

Matt, on the other hand, picked me up and took me out to go dancing. That suited me just fine. You can picture me wearing short boots and a mini-skirt, fashionable in the 1980's. We had a lot of fun dancing, but didn't find as much to talk about. Matt was handsome and friendly, but a little quieter than Andy.

As the weeks advanced, I went to a Christian concert with Andy and another couple whom he knew well; I discovered that I really liked his friends. Matt and I went out to eat. I hadn't seen any point in mentioning to either Matt or Andy that I was dating someone else, too, because this was casual

---

* The name has been changed.

and there was no commitment. However, on the Friday after Thanksgiving I received anonymous red roses from one of them at my workplace. There was a poem but no name:

To she who must work today,
From him who must not;
Since I cannot be with you,
Let these roses take my place.

Whom would I thank, and how would I find out which one sent them? This could get me into trouble! I knew Andy was away on a trip. Matt was coming over to take me out, so I brought the roses to my apartment and set them in a prominent place near the door. When Matt arrived, I figured he'd see them and take credit if he'd sent them. If he didn't say anything, I wouldn't either, and I'd assume that they weren't from him. Matt arrived and took one look at the roses. "Who sent you those?" he asked. "It must have been a nicer guy than me." Wow! So they were from Andy! How romantic!

I was starting to lean toward Andy, but the next two dates made it clear. Matt was a super-nice guy, easy-going, likeable, and fairly athletic, which were all a great fit for me. He didn't have a particularly strong personality, though, and sometimes I felt like my strengths could overwhelm him. Andy, on the other hand, wanted a girlfriend who was intelligent and who had strong opinions. He liked to debate, argue, and discuss issues, and he said he enjoyed my capacity to disagree with him! Matt valued calm, but Andy valued some turbulence.

Andy was a stronger leader, as well. In two parallel dates, Matt and I and two of my friends went to downtown Detroit to see a play. Matt let me drive to the Fisher Theater— he was absolutely no help at navigating, and he let me pay for the tickets. My friends cautioned me that they didn't think that he was a great fit for me. By contrast, Andy took me to Detroit to Greek Town and the North American Auto Show. He drove in the city and he was an awesome navigator. He told me about taking groups of students to Germany and getting them on planes and trains all over Europe in the summers. He seemed very confident and strong. By this date, some definite chemistry was developing between us.

I explained to Matt that I was not able to see him any longer, and I told Andy that I would not see anybody else so that we could determine whether we were right for each other. As we dated, I began to fall in love with Andy, and he with me. My heart said, "yes," but my mind still had objections. Andy was not particularly athletic, but I pursued sports whole-heartedly, and that difference between us was a source of tension. To his credit, though, he tried to join me in my love for all things active. He had determined that he would do whatever it took to win my heart. I later learned that his mom and sister were astonished and amused, seeing him leave the house carrying ice-skates for a date with me. Apparently, he'd never skated before in his life! He tried cross-country skiing, falling down countless times but jumping back up so fast that I wasn't really sure that I'd seen him go down. He bought a bike and we rode together.

Still, Andy was an academic at heart; he read books, wrote articles, and maintained a large collection of books and CDs. He really preferred to spend the day reading and relaxing, while I preferred to spend a day being active. I had always pictured myself marrying someone who was athletic and constantly "on the go" like me. I really wondered how we would work out our differences. I spent time praying about this, asking for God's guidance. Andy's faith was important to him, too, and he sought God's leading as well. Ultimately, God led us toward each other. God knew my future—He knew what I would need in a spouse more than I did! Andy treated me better than any guy ever had, and I think his kindness and character won me over. In 1989, we became engaged to be married.

During the next few months, we were busy with wedding plans. However, that wasn't the only thing going on. In March of 1990, we were sitting at a dinner theater, and suddenly I felt pain in my low back. The pain traveled down my right leg; it was so cramping and uncomfortable that we left early, even though we'd made plans with friends for later.

For the next three months, I saw my primary care doctor and continued working, although I decreased my hours to four-day weeks, taking Wednesdays off to rest my back. We continued with wedding preparations, but the pain frightened me. It wasn't getting worse, but it wasn't getting better, either. I knew genetically I was at risk for back problems, having inherited mild scoliosis from my mother's family and a tendency toward disc problems from my father. I had also experienced back pain before, after an injury during one of my physical therapy internships. A three-hundred-pound patient had fallen while I was walking next to him, holding a "gait training belt" around his waist. When he started to go down, I'd lowered him to the floor to help break his fall. That's what my classmates and I were trained to do in physical therapy school. My back was very sore afterwards, but the pain had lasted only a weekend. Then I was back to normal, or so I thought. There had been a few more isolated weekends of back pain related to my work, but the pain always went away. Besides, I'd always taken care of my back, keeping fit and using good posture and lifting techniques.

Getting Married:
A Disability Begins as Pain Becomes a Monster

The week before our wedding, my back pain became disabling. I had seen two orthopedic surgeons in a twenty-four hour period, looking for answers. The pain had actually been aggravated by their examinations. The next day when I bent forward in the shower, I felt something tear behind my right hip. The pain which had begun three months earlier and had allowed me to work 80% of full-time got dramatically worse. It now exploded into my life as an all-consuming fire. I couldn't sit, I couldn't walk more than about a block, and the only semi-comfortable position was lying down. Going to work was out of the question. This really was frightening. What was happening to me?

The day before our wedding, I called my doctor's office and spoke to a nurse. After describing my back and leg pain and the severity of my symptoms, she advised me to go to the emergency room. "I can't," I replied. "I'm getting married tomorrow." Everything from the church to the photographer to the reception hall was reserved and pre-arranged, and my family had flown and driven in from around the country. I wasn't going to interrupt my wedding for diagnostic tests or whatever the Emergency Room would want me to do. In fact, going anywhere right now would only make things worse.

July 7, 1990, the day of our wedding, arrived. I canceled

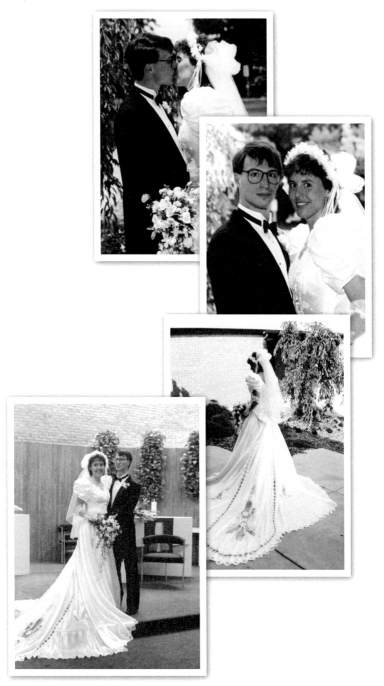

My wedding day. Smiling through the pain. Great joy and great pain coincide. It's astonishing to me that the pain doesn't show.

my hair appointment 30 minutes away. My wonderful sister-in-law Sharon quickly arranged my hair for me at my apartment. We drove to the church where my sister Barb helped me put on my wedding gown. It was beautiful white satin with pearls on the bodice and a four-foot train. I wore flats because heels were off-limits with back pain. My father walked me down the aisle, talking to me to distract me from my pain and nervousness, but I didn't hear a word he said! All I wanted to do was see Andy and hang on to him for dear life. During his sermon, my dad teared up as he spoke to us. It was as if he had a premonition that back pain was going to be a significant part of our married life together. Dad was impressed with and grateful to Andy for his commitment and care for me. After Dad's sermon, we exchanged personalized vows and our rings. Wow. We were married now! What a relief. *I had done it.*

Then came the receiving line. Andy and I were elated that we were married, and it was wonderful to greet our guests. But the pain was building, burning, growing, and we still had to pose for pictures. I desperately needed to lie down for an hour, so a sheet was spread on the floor in a quiet room where I laid down in my wedding gown. I did some deep breathing and tried to relax. These wedding pictures were going to last a lifetime. I didn't want to see pain on my face when I looked at them for years to come, so I smiled through the pain. *I was learning that great pain and great joy can be present simultaneously in life.*

After the pictures we went on to the reception—a brief event including lunch and cutting/serving the cake. There was a pianist, but fortunately we hadn't hired a band, so no dancing was expected. I sat through the meal, secretly miserable. The 800 mg. of Ibuprofen I was taking every four hours was not even touching my pain. I finally retreated to the ladies' room where I gingerly lowered myself to lying on the couch and dissolved into tears. That was it; I'd had it! The pain overwhelmed me. I wondered later whether the wedding guests who'd stumbled across me in the women's bathroom thought I regretted getting married. It wasn't that at all; I simply couldn't cope with any more pain in one day.

We reluctantly canceled our honeymoon to the Canadian Rockies. Our plane tickets into Calgary, our reservations in Banff and Lake Louise, and our tickets to the Calgary Rodeo went unused. Instead, we spent a few quiet days by Lake Michigan. It wasn't much of a honeymoon, and physical intimacy was difficult at best. We were deeply disappointed, but we tried to make the best of it. When we returned to Ann Arbor, I spent the first ten weeks of our marriage on bed rest except for my doctor's appointments, diagnostic tests, and physical therapy. Instead of being the physical therapist, wearing the white lab coat, I was now the physical therapy patient. After the ten-week period I tried to return to work, but I could only work two hours, every other day. *I knew I was in more pain than any of the patients I was treating.* After three months of trying to increase my hours with minimal improvement, I was advised by a physician to quit working. I filed for short-term disability and left the work world for life at home—at least for now.

My sense of displacement was immense. I had worked so hard through college and two years of graduate school to become a physical therapist, and I loved my career. Now I had a mere two to three hours out of bed per day and no good explanations of what was causing my severe pain. The doctors ordered a number of diagnostic tests. A CT scan and an MRI revealed moderately bulging discs in my lower back. A myelogram was done where dye was injected into my back to show what was happening to the nerves coming off the spinal cord. EMG testing was performed to measure the nerve signal strength reaching my leg muscles. Both tests showed some damage to nerves leading to my right leg. But my test results could not explain the severity of my pain, and treatments did little to alleviate it. I tried aquatherapy with little progress, but at least I could stand up in the swimming pool and move around a little. I continued to consult physicians, but none felt I was a good surgical candidate. My life as I'd known it had come to a screeching halt.

I felt betrayed by my body. I felt like I was in free fall, hurtling down into a deep black pit with nothing to break my fall. I felt abandoned by modern medicine, which seemed to have an answer for so many medical problems but not for mine. No one knew how to help me; I seemed beyond rescue.

There was a very tall plant in our apartment, which grew as high as the ceiling. It looked like it belonged in a jungle. As I stared at that plant, day after day, it came to symbolize my former life, fully developed and with many large, hand-sized leaves. "Chop that plant down!" I directed Andy when he came home from teaching one day. "My old life is gone! I want you to chop down the plant, because I've lost all of that!" Andy reflected a moment, and then he did chop the plant off, close to the dirt. We both watched as the eight foot stalk came crashing down into the room. I began to cry. I cried and cried, pouring out all my frustration, grief, and anger at losing my ability to work, play sports, and travel. Each leaf on that plant symbolized something I had lost: tennis, golfing, flying on a plane, hiking in the mountains, working as a physical therapist, and sitting to eat meals. Now I was having to eat most meals while lying on the floor. There had been leaves representing running, biking, canoeing down a river; leaves for church activities and cross-country skiing and much, much more. All that was left of the plant now were roots and a stump. I stared at it through my lens of sadness and loss.

What Once Was A Healthy Spine

The healthy spine is made up of vertebrae (bones) and discs (soft tissue) between the vertebrae. The discs separate and cushion the bones. There are seven small vertebrae and discs in the cervical spine (neck); twelve in the thoracic spine (rib-cage area); and five large vertebrae and thicker discs in the lumbar spine (low back). Beneath the lumbar spine is the sacrum, a triangular-shaped bone which has no discs, since it is composed of several bones fused together.

Vertebrae are named according to an alphanumeric system: C1 is the highest vertebra in the neck, or cervical spine; C2 is the second highest. T1 is the highest bone in the thoracic region, and L1 the highest lumbar vertebra. The disc is named for the vertebrae above and below it: the L1-2 disc is the disc between the first and second lumbar vertebra. The L4-5 disc is between the two lowest lumbar vertebrae.

It is important to have healthy discs, because they do the job of absorbing shock and also allowing movement in the spine between vertebrae. Without discs, it would be impossible for your spine to absorb shock or to bend in any direction! The normal disc is roughly oval-shaped with a convex front and a concave back. The center of the disc, called the nucleus, is

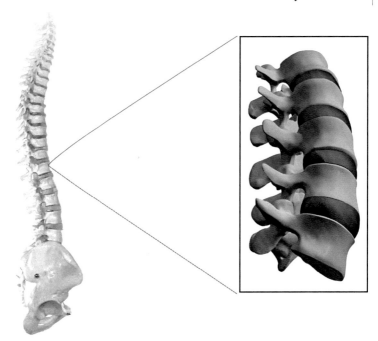

The Human Spine with lumbar spine enlargement.

soft like jelly. The nucleus is surrounded by rings, called the annulus, which are of a more solid consistency. In a normal, healthy disc, the nucleus acts like a fluid-filled cushion which can be loaded and can absorb shock. Imagine it as a tire filled with Jello, or a jelly-filled donut. The annular rings (like the tire) need to be tough yet flexible.

As a disc degenerates through aging or injury, the annulus begins to crack or tear from the inside rings outward. At this early stage, healing is often possible. As the cracks deepen, however, the nucleus travels outward into the cracks. The Jello moves outward into the tire, or the jelly moves out into the donut. These cracks can be painful, because the disc is connected to small nerve fibers which can sense pain. At this stage, the disc can already start to bulge. When the crack is completely torn through, the outer rings of the annulus can bulge further or even rupture backward, and the fluid of the nucleus can leak out backward. This is a painful condition, and very hard to heal, because the disc does not have a direct blood supply. As a disc degenerates, it can also become thinner, causing people to get shorter as they age. The thin disc does a poor job of separating the vertebra above from the vertebra below it.

Directly behind the discs, traveling through a vertical canal of bone, is the spinal cord. It runs from the brain to the tail bone. At each level of the spinal cord, there are medium-sized nerves called "nerve roots" coming off to the side. The nerve roots carry nerve signals to and from the arms and legs. When a disc bulges backward, it can put pressure on the nerve root behind it, causing pain to be "referred" down the arm or leg. A thin disc can also indirectly cause pain in a nerve root because the upper vertebra and the lower vertebra do not have enough room between them for the nerve roots to come out without being pinched.

The vertebrae also have "facet joints" behind them, which help guide movement. Projections of bone reach up or down to link with the projections of bone from the neighboring vertebra. Where they meet, the facet joint forms. This can also be a source of pain if these become inflamed or arthritic.

What I Think Happened to Me

My own theory: Early in life the discs have a large percentage of water; aging dehydrates them. The earlier in life the disc tears, the more painful it is, because a torn hydrated disc gets more inflamed than a torn dehydrated disc. The inflammation causes pressure pain from excess fluid, like a thumb throbbing after being hit by a hammer. The inflammation process also brings painful chemicals to the area of injury to try to help heal it. The goal is healing, but the chemicals can actually make the pain worse. This is my theory for why my discs are so painful. Since my pain started so young at age twenty-seven, my discs weren't dehydrated yet. I believe that they are chronically inflamed.

There is a sharp contrast between the abstract biological description of my disc problems and the shattering effect they had on my life.

It's not easy being in a rare category. My type of disc pain is less common than the more typical disc degeneration with dehydration. My torn discs produce severe pain, which is more disabling than average. So sometimes I am compared to people who can still sit or stand or work despite their disc problems—leaving me to feel as if I've failed somehow. There was a lot of pressure to fit into norms for back problems—have physical therapy for a few weeks, and return to work—and the fact that my condition was outside of those norms made it very difficult to explain to others. It was very difficult to understand ourselves!

CHAPTER TWO

The Beginning of My Horizontal Life

My Life Within Four Walls:
Mourning the Life I Once Had

My broad life narrows down as if its activities have been forced through a funnel. Crowding and jostling for position, the traits of strength are squeezed out. Only the weakness seems to trickle through. All of a sudden, my active life of working, golfing, and running is gone, replaced by resting, confinement, and persistent pain. My daily routine is repetitive and rigid: wake up, shower, get dressed; eat breakfast lying on the floor, and begin lying down on the day bed until lunch. Get up, eat quickly, do a few exercises, stand for several minutes, then lie down on the day bed for the afternoon. Wait for Andy to come home from teaching.

Forget commuting to work in my sporty red Mazda coup

with a sunroof. Forget treating patients and enjoying the process of helping them get better. Forget being part of a vibrant clinic with stimulating colleagues. The clock becomes an enemy, every tick-tock a reminder of the way time—which used to fly—now crawls through the day. In our small apartment, the view of the four walls quickly grows stale. The beige paint and beige curtains and beige carpet mirror the monotony of a never-changing environment. My eyes seek color and art like a parched man seeks water.

The pain itself makes me feel nervous and insecure. I don't like it, and I don't want it to stay. My body has always given me the pleasure of movement and strength; now it's giving me this distressing input of pain, around the clock. My back is throbbing like a thumb after being struck by a hammer — struck over and over again. My right leg hurts so much I can't even stand having the weight of the bed covers on it. I've had pain before, like menstrual cramps or an occasional headache, but this pain is in a different league. It makes me want to panic. I'm feeling desperate to get rid of it. But how?

Evenings aren't bad, because I'm with Andy. We talk and read and watch TV together. Every morning, though, he goes off to work with the rest of the world. The apartment building grows quiet and the parking lot empties out. I feel abandoned as everyone goes off to their jobs. I've always had somewhere to go, too: either school or work. Now everything's changed. Each morning the question of how to pass the time resurfaces, taunting and heckling me like a circus clown gone insane. Everyone likes an occasional day off, but being an invalid for weeks that turn into months? I don't have a clue how to live this way. What do you do with your days when you can't "do" very much? How do you adjust when everything you're used to is taken away? Reading becomes an escape ... for a while ... listening to talk radio ... watching TV news ... renting movies ... but deep in my soul, there is a need to create, to exert my mark on the environment; a need to do more than passively consume modern media. Victory over the taunting question of how to spend time demands an active response, so I write in my journal and find a bit of relief.

Redefining myself and my purpose are crucial. What is the meaning of my life now? How long will I be like this? Can I survive with these limitations? Any time I am creating something instead of just surviving another day, my life seems bearable. So I begin painting t-shirts and small ceramic houses while lying down. It seems important to have something each day that I've accomplished, some tiny sign of productivity to show for it. Only an hour or two a day of so-called "work" is possible, but over weeks and months, that hour might become significant and have power.

My friends come over, but they don't know what to do with me; we always did such active things, and now all we can do is hang out and talk. I can see their restlessness to get outside and do something. I feel like I'm boring them. My bike sits vacant, currently functioning as something on which to hang clothes. Cross-country skis peek out from the closet, and my tennis racket hangs forlornly from a hook. I've got to get my mind on something else! I need a mental challenge, a goal, so I begin studying German since Andy is a German teacher. I try to enter his world. He begins to tutor me in the evenings.

I also spend time praying. It never occurred to me before that prayer gives people dignity, that it empowers people in humble circumstances, but now I discover that it does. Joining thoughts with God in some mysterious way to help impact His work in the world is an incredible privilege. This is especially true for someone who is otherwise marginalized from society. I've always been too busy to do much of this. I start to pray for every sick or lonely person I know. I pray for the homeless shelters and free medical clinics in my town and county. I pray for mission work going on around the world. Some people I know have started a short-term missions group that sends teams of people to developing countries for one to two weeks. The teams distribute eyeglasses, provide dental care, or work on construction projects to serve the poor. I get a schedule of the teams and pray for their safe travel and that many poor people will be helped. In the quiet of the apartment, spending time alone with God in prayer, the presence of God seems palpable. At times I can sense Him in the room with me, and I don't feel quite so alone.

Andy and I are visited by Lloyd Stuhr who did our marriage counseling. Rather than let the relationship fade away, Lloyd sticks by us and begins to visit us weekly at our apartment. He seems to know how lost we feel. He encourages us to focus outward, to entertain the unexpected possibility that God might use my suffering to help others who suffer. Lloyd recommends that I meet with a Stephen Minister, a woman from our church who has been trained to provide peer support and Christian care. So Deb Scobel comes into our lives. She shows up every week to listen as I pour out my emotions to her. Deb is very caring, patient, and encouraging, and her commitment to me helps me feel valued.

I'm wrestling with uncertainty, and I have many questions. What does this pain mean for me? How can I make plans now? I'm so used to planning my life a few months at a time. This pain and disability put everything in jeopardy. I'm forced to guess about whether I will or won't be able to work again, how and where we'll spend the holidays, even whether or not we'll be able to have children. People around us are always making plans, projecting their lives into the future. What happens when you can't anymore? I know other people's plans are subject to change or cancellation, too, but they at least have the illusion of having some control over their lives. I feel totally powerless over the future or what will happen.

As for the plant which Andy chopped down, he continues to water the stump, leaving the pot by the window. I simply ignore it. After several weeks, though, to my surprise, the plant begins to send up a new shoot from its old stump. The roots must still be living and active. A few weeks later the shoot starts to grow a single leaf resembling the old leaves, but new. As I watch its progress, I begin to think that a new life might be possible for me. Gradually, as the weeks turn into months, I start to understand that if God gives me my life back, this is how He might do it. It won't happen all at once, and it won't be the same life as before. Gradually, however, He might grow my life back: one leaf at a time, one ability at a time, one relationship at a time.

What does it mean that the roots of my life are still the same as before? My ability to think and use my mind is still present, if not my ability to use my body fully. My personality is basically unchanged, my faith in God is intact, and there are still people in my life who love me and whom I love. I need to be patient and give this process the time that it needs ... and I may need to accept that the pain won't go away. I don't like it at all but perhaps it is enough to go on...to find meaning and purpose in a life of pain that I would never choose but has come to me anyway.

My Stephen Minister, Deb Scobel, gives me this quote from the Bible to think about:

> "For I know the plans I have for you," declares the Lord. "Plans to prosper you and not to harm you, plans to give you hope and a future" (Jeremiah 29:11).

Even though I don't know my own future, this verse says God has plans for me. He wants to prosper me, not harm me. He wants to give me hope. This verse is comforting whenever I remember it. It stretches my faith, because I can't depend on myself any longer; I need to depend more fully on God. My inner battle is between having faith and having fear.

Trying to deal with that inner battle is hard work; I am very aware that my faith is not steady, but that it vacillates. I vacillate between having faith that God is in control and will take care of me, and being overwhelmed with fear that my life has been irreversibly changed and will never be the same as it was. I fear that I won't be able to cope with a life of pain. I fear that having been struck down, I will be destroyed.

It's only when I remember that God really loves me that the fears recede. It's only when I think about the way God has touched my life that I have confidence. I remind myself that my church family has "been there" for me, that my husband still loves me, and that I can find encouraging Bible verses like Jeremiah 29:11 (above). These are all ways that God's touch is active and reaching into my life and into my troubled thoughts. True, I have doubts, which come and go, and my faith is not steady, but that's ok. God accepts me just the way I am, doubts, fears, and all. He'll keep reaching into my life to help me learn to lean on Him, learn to follow His lead, and learn to receive from Him. He'll help me find my way in this entirely new, narrow life I have.

Lament

Oh, God,
I'm so scared
My life has come apart
And I can't put it back together.

I feel like a turtle that's been flipped on its back
Helpless—Vulnerable
Won't you come to me and help?

I cry every day now
It used to be quite rare
I'm trapped in this pain nightmare
Oh, God, don't you care?

I know You are powerful
You created the universe
You know my body cell by cell
Just say the word, and You can make me well.

Or lead me to the right doctors
You are wise and I need wisdom:
To choose the right treatments;
Navigate the medical system
So my disabling pain will be relieved.

I know You've promised never to leave me
But You feel so far away
I know You walk with me through suffering
But my heart's cry is to be well.

Please don't leave me in this condition, Lord
I don't want to stay this way

My dreams are too big for this narrow life.

Describing Pain

At its worst, my pain is harsh, cruel, and raw. It's a cramping, throbbing, burning scorpion's sting deep within. It's a rotten companion, selfish, and mean. If pain were an emotion, it would feel like what you sense the moment a lion's claw gashes your skin: anger and fear all mixed up together. Pain wields its power without mercy or care for the damage inflicted ... as the viper which strikes coldly and suddenly. An unwelcome visitor, it shows up without invitation and stays as long as it wants. Pain is a thief, stealing function and canceling plans—never apologizing or making amends. It offers no promise of a better future, only challenges its victim to a game of survival.

Can you cope with daily pain and the depression that always attends it? Can you learn how to struggle against self-pity, bitterness, and envy toward others who don't have pain? Can you learn to cry and wail and let out some of the emotional pain, or will it drive you to make self-destructive choices? And where is God, a loving God, if He allows this pain into your life?

My pain is less in the morning and worsens as the day progresses. This is such a familiar pattern: I live for mornings and I think of the afternoons and evenings as my harder times. They are almost always a mandatory rest time for me. I'm Cinderella, only my coach turns into a pumpkin at noon instead of midnight. Occasionally, maybe once every other month, my pain withdraws and allows an unexpected good day to appear, and I breathe deeply and freely again! It recedes so unpredictably, though, that plans can't be made to use the unaccustomed function. Too precious to waste on an "average" day, the longing is to have a celebration event—a wedding, a party, a family reunion, a holiday—on which to spend the rationed function. It's such a relief to have ease of body and mind.

But the celebration events are seldom on good days. Pain is no respecter of special days and seems to rear its ugly head in unusually cruel ways on those "celebration" days. The cobra slithers in once again.

Pain is a charging bull, and I'm trapped in the bullpen with it. I'd like to be the toreador, fighting directly against the bull, but pain can't be fought head-on. Unlike the bullfighter, who waves a red flag to get the bull's attention, I try to make the bull lose interest in me. I wear subdued colors and quiet my movements. I try to stay out of the bull's line of sight. I test him with my carefully-chosen activities to see how he responds. If he notices me, he might ignore me. If he becomes angry enough, however, he charges me, and I have to drop to the ground. I lie down as he comes at me, hoping he will stop the charge and assume I'm "dead." After I lie down for several hours or days, he wanders off. I might be able to get up for a while, but I can never leave the pen. The bull is always close by.

Pain drives me inward, as it demands my attention, like a whining toddler inside my brain. At times it screams at me and all other input is blocked out. At other times it's a dull chatter, a nagging aggravation. It narrows my world and changes my goals. I no longer strive for pleasure or adventure, but put focus into cessation of movement and careful positioning, so the pain can quiet down to a tolerable level. I feel fragile, vulnerable, as shatter-prone as crystal.

Paul and Helen

The symbolism of the plant helped me to experience hope. One of the new leaves/relationships which was growing was with my in-laws, Paul and Helen Smith. They were dear people who accepted me immediately into their family after Andy asked me to marry him. We had gotten engaged when Andy took me away for the weekend to a surprise destination: Point Pelee in Canada. It was a peninsula of land stretching south into Lake Erie, with boardwalks through marshes and wooded areas for hiking and enjoying the scenery.

Andy asked me to marry him on the beach at the tip of the peninsula, and I said yes. He let out a yell, "yah-hoo!" which could be heard up and down the beach. We were so much in love, we just floated through the rest of that day. The next day, we returned to Ann Arbor, where Andy gave me a diamond ring. Then we went straight to his parent's house. Paul and Helen were home, and as we walked into the living room, I held my hand forward so that they could see the diamond sparkling. Helen shouted, "I knew it! I knew it!" and she ran around the room giving high-five's and hugs to everyone. What a reception! Paul, the quieter of the two, grinned and hugged us.

Over the next months, Helen helped me shop for my wedding dress. We got to know each other as we went from one bridal shop to the next, and we were together when I finally tried on the perfect gown. As we looked at each other in the mirror, our eyes met, and we both smiled. There was no doubt: it was the one. From the beginning, Helen was a friend, and we enjoyed each other's company very much.

Paul and Helen's graciousness became very apparent after the wedding when my back pain had become so disabling. Initially, all of us thought I would improve with treatment, return to work, and get on with life. As the months wore on, however, treatments proved to be of only limited value. My trial return to work failed, and we began to realize that this back problem might become a bigger part of our married life than anticipated. Naturally, we were all disappointed, but Paul and Helen never said a word of that to us other than in supportive, empathetic ways. They could have had regrets that their only son married a woman with disabling pain; they could have expressed disappointment with me, but they never did.

The summer after we got married, Andy had to take a group of students to Germany for several weeks as part of his job. Since I was still very limited by pain, I was unable to live alone while he was gone. I couldn't shop for groceries or lift them. I tried doing some light shopping, but my pain would be so severe I'd be hanging on the checkout counter, leaning forward and pushing down with my arms, trying to "unload" my spine. Even trying to lift or bring a few groceries into the house, or to stand more than a few minutes at the kitchen counter to prepare food, caused me agony. Trying to lift wet clothes out of the washing machine was out of the question. So I stayed with Paul and Helen for two weeks, and I lay on their floor as the days went by, because sitting was so painful.

For their part, Andy's parents never said or did anything to make me feel uncomfortable; their acceptance of me never wavered. It was awkward and humbling for me, after having a college education and career, to be dependent upon my in-laws and unable to do much at all to help them, but they made it seem almost normal. Paul and Helen showed me hospitality and loved me as a daughter, much as they loved their own daughter Jenny. They refused to hold me at arm's length as a disabled daughter-in-law who disappointed their hopes for their son. Helen helped me see that even if I never regained a normal life, she valued me for the love I'd brought into Andy's life. She appreciated me for my place in relationships, not just for what I could or couldn't do. Helen and Paul were disappointed for me and Andy, because they knew my pain made our lives harder, but never in me. Is it any wonder, then, that I loved them for it?

Helen enjoyed sewing, and she had remnants of fabric from the many dresses and shirts she'd made for Jenny and Andy over the years. She brought out these pieces of brightly colored cloth and suggested that I make a quilt. I was willing to try almost anything rather than lie passively on the floor for hours on end; that was so demeaning and demoralizing. So I started cutting five-inch squares from my prone position, and she told me stories about Andy and Jenny when they were young. The fabric remnants sparked her memories of other times and places, and I began to get a more complete sense of the family history.

I could only cut squares for about an hour before my neck and shoulders protested; everything is more difficult to do lying down. The project was something life-giving, though, because it pointed to the future. A quilt always does that: who knows how it will be used, and by whom? At the same time, it tied me into the family's past. As I listened to Helen's stories, which broadened to include her childhood memories, I became part of the family fabric. It gave me an appreciation for the oral legends of the family which I could begin to carry forward. I had always "done life" by achieving things, doing things, making things. Helen was subtly leading me into a new way of life, which was to discover and appreciate what others had done or accomplished or achieved, and to value those stories and pass them on.

Later that year, when it came time to sew the quilt, I could only sit at the sewing machine fifteen minutes a day. At first, it frustrated me terribly to have to limit myself to that, because I thought at that pace I'd never get done. I was so restless and impatient, I hated quitting just as I felt that I was getting started. Over time, however, the quilt took shape, and after six weeks of fifteen minutes a day, it was finished. Like the story of the tortoise and the hare, significant things could be accomplished by someone moving slowly. I much preferred being the hare, moving at blinding speed, but the tortoise that I had become was only going to function at a slow and steady pace. According to the author of that children's story, at least sometimes, "slow and steady wins the race."

Mayo Clinic and Pain Clinic

After Andy returned from Germany that summer, we made the decision to travel to the Mayo Clinic in Rochester, Minnesota. We had spent the first year searching for a diagnosis in southeastern Michigan. I had gone to see twenty doctors and had multiple diagnostic tests. We chose Mayo Clinic because we had heard of their team approach. In theory, specialists would confer with each other about my case and hopefully be able to solve the mystery of what was causing my pain. I was assigned an appointment in October, but we chose to go earlier, in July, because that's when Andy had time off from teaching. So we arrived without an appointment, and as a result I was assigned to a physician in Gastroenterology, who then referred me to Neurology.

The largest building of the clinic was designed with multiple stories for various specialties. In the center of each floor was a large waiting room (NO WINDOWS) where patients spent hours or days waiting to hear their names called over the microphone. Of course, the assumption was that patients could sit for hours or days waiting for the right moment to come, but I couldn't sit. Andy dutifully packed a foam mat with pillows and carried it to the appropriate floor so I could lie down on the carpet and wait. This was unusual, so I endured many questioning glances, and I felt unsafe being in the way of foot traffic. We spent two weeks doing this, being referred next to Oncology to rule out cancer of the spine or pelvis. While waiting, it helped to make small talk with the other patients. We realized that other people were caught in health quagmires, too. Mayo Clinic was a place where many people came, driven by the same blend of hope and desperation that we experienced.

I remember lying in an MRI tube for the third time. The Mayo Clinic wanted its own diagnostic tests. Inside that tube, amid the racket of the magnets, it seemed to be just me and God. I was praying urgently, begging God to lead the doctors to a correct diagnosis and treatment, even if it meant surgery. I could become healthy and strong again, return to work, and maybe even try to have a baby. I desperately longed to have my ability to stand, sit, and function restored. Wouldn't my life be more useful to God and others if I were well? Beyond being useful, it just would be such a relief to be rid of constant pain! I wanted my normal life back; it was so much easier and so much more gratifying than this awful life of being sidelined by disabling pain.

We finally met with a neurosurgeon after two-and-a-half weeks at the clinic. Based on the test results at the time, he and the other physicians I'd seen were unable to add anything to the diagnosis of degenerative disc disease. He said I was not a surgical candidate, so I would have to learn to live with disabling pain. He made the blanket statement which I don't think any doctor should normally say: that nothing could be done medically to help me. His words thundered through me. I shuddered as the door to hope inside my mind slammed shut. There was a deafening roar.

The blackness of that moment, and the lurch of despair and hopelessness deep inside me were overwhelming. I broke down and wept. I limped out of his office with Andy's help, leaning on a cane because of the radiating pain in my right leg, and the surgeon watched me go. He had to have wondered what was wrong with me and why he couldn't figure out my case. He should have said that he didn't have any answers, but that modern medicine is always making new discoveries. They might have something in the future to help me. He didn't have the right to take away all hope.

To me, the search for answers to my pain seemed like being lost in a very long maze, unable to find my way out. Which direction do I turn next? Have I already been here before? How long will I be trapped in this maze? Is there anyone who has the knowledge and skill to help me get out? After being screened by a psychiatrist, we returned to Ann Arbor, where I was referred to one of the several pain clinics in southeastern Michigan.

If I had any hopes of this helping to ease my adjustment into living with pain, I was to be disappointed. For nine months I followed their program set by a comprehensive team of anesthesiology, physical therapy, social work, and psychology. The epidural steroid injections provided short-term pain relief (two to three weeks), but every time I increased function, my pain would flare, sending me into a downward spiral of relapse.

The same was true for physical therapy. The treatments of traction, mobilizations, stretching, and strengthening would give me tiny increases in function until I reached some imperceptible limit, and my progress would all come crashing down around me again. How could five minutes of walking on a treadmill be okay one day, and six, seven, and eight minutes in incremental treatments be safe, but the day we reached ten minutes of walking cause a flare-up of excruciating pain and muscle spasms*? What kind of a back problem did I have, that

---

*A guideline for physical therapy is that it may increase pain for several hours or a day after treatment, due to tissue manipulation. However, the pain should be back to normal or improved by twenty-four hours post-treatment...thirty-six hours at the longest. There should be a lessening of pain overall over the course of several treatments. Physical therapy goals are usually to decrease swelling, increase normal motion, decrease pain, and increase strength.

it was so reactive and inflammatory, and the pain so severe?

It was as if I had a raw egg instead of discs inside my spine, and my mission was to avoid breaking it. How does one live carefully enough not to break an egg? I was unaccustomed to this degree of fragility.

The psychological aspects of treatment were no more helpful. I was instructed by a "pain psychologist" to read a book on Zen Buddhism. The book explained if I were only less goal-oriented, less "type A," perhaps my pain would lessen or become more tolerable. I should picture myself as an archer who cared little for whether or not he hit a target or a bull's eye with his arrow. My understanding of Buddhism was that it asks a person to empty him or herself of desires and goals in order to avoid suffering. However, in the presence of pain, I didn't want to empty myself. I wanted to fill myself with God's presence, and with all that He could bring, to help me handle the pain. In the presence of pain, I chose to retain goals. I was not a person who could accept not caring about my accomplishments, my relationships, or my future.

Zen Buddhism did not reduce my pain; moreover, it seemed to ask me to give up what I had left: my dreams, my hopes, my goals. I wanted to choose an active response, not a passive one. It was so frustrating to be directed this way, after so many months of effort in the pain clinic, that I became angry. The fact that my discs were degenerating and that there was physical damage to my tissue was not being acknowledged or validated. It seemed to me that the psychologist at the pain clinic was implying that the problem was my attitude. If it were a case of mind over matter—well, my mind said that matter mattered. I came home, and for the first time in my life, I was so angry and disappointed that I had to smash something. I grabbed a water bottle and threw it across the room. It hit the wall and broke, spraying water everywhere.

Andy stood there speechless, awestruck by my powerful display of emotions. After a pause, he came over and put his arms around me as I dissolved into tears. He rubbed my back consolingly and murmured, "If I had to endure everything you're going through, I'd feel the same way you do. Your pain is not the result of being 'type A;' you didn't do anything to bring this upon yourself. This is not your fault. You're doing everything you can to get well."

Andy continued, "That psychologist seems to delight in contradicting both your personality and your beliefs. He seems really ignorant of the fact that you have tissue damage. He doesn't have anything to offer you; he's doing more harm than good."

We agreed that we were done with that particular pain clinic.

Misfortune Cookies

Life had gotten so strange and bizarre; Andy used the term "Kafkaesque" to describe dealing with the medical system. In Kafka's books, there is usually a character who is being punished or treated as though he were a criminal. He is never told what his crime is, however, or why he's being treated the way he is. In our case, what we had always experienced with health matters was now turned on its head. Whenever one of us had gotten sick, we'd simply gone to a doctor, he or she would prescribe a medication, and we'd get well again. This time the medical system was letting us down and not providing any helpful answers.

I had been to over twenty physicians in southeastern Michigan, who worked in half a dozen different hospital systems. The Mayo Clinic in Minnesota had been a seventh, and then we had returned to Michigan to a pain clinic there: an eighth. Each new system required a multi-page form to be filled out, which was no problem. They also required a physical examination including the straight-leg raise test though, which was a problem. In this test, I had to lie down on my back, and the doctor raised my leg as high in the air as it could go. It always made my symptoms worse, and not just a little worse. Having the straight-leg raise test done caused terrific cramping and nerve pain in my leg which made my life miserable for several weeks afterward. Doctors refused to omit this test, irrespective of our reasons. I didn't understand why they wouldn't listen to me. I didn't understand why they refused to believe what I said would happen if they did that. What did I know? I was just the lowly patient, and they were the all-powerful doctors. Their inability to listen caused serious harm.

There were multiple CT scans, X-rays, MRIs, and other diagnostic tests. Countless hours had been spent in waiting rooms and in numerous exam rooms, nervously waiting for the new physician to walk in the door.

Andy's experience of dealing with the large medical systems was that you get shuffled from one person to another with little information. You're not even sure why you're being sent from one professional to another, and it's a big, impersonal bureaucracy. Andy and I were surprised at how each new physician disregarded anything that had been learned to date. The prevalent policy of starting over with each patient and refusing to accept diagnostic tests done anywhere else struck us as wasteful and unnecessarily arduous. The legal climate in which doctors function dictated some of this, but it seemed to us that physicians' egos were responsible as well.

Patients are labeled if they "doctor hop," yet surgeons typically select the "safest" patients from the new group they see each month. They can easily pass along the unusual patients to the next doctor. So a person with chronic pain can be seeking help, cooperating with the system, enduring repeated diagnostic tests and painful exams, and really get nowhere. They can obtain a negative label, "doctor hopper", even though they're doing everything they've been asked to do. They've been compliant patients, but aren't recognized for it.

Patients also have to deal with the very real stigma associated with chronic pain. Because pain is invisible, there are some who doubt that chronic pain is real, or who doubt that it can be disabling. Some physicians believe that patients with chronic pain could get well if they pushed themselves through the pain. "No pain, no gain" is perhaps appropriate for strength training a muscle, but it's not appropriate for disc pain, ligament injuries, or joint problems. In these cases, pushing through pain can cause very real tissue damage.

There is a theory which suggests that chronic pain continues after the tissue heals, because of changes in the nervous system. Patients are told that their injury has healed after a time period between six weeks and six months post-injury. In my opinion, this is an overly simplistic view of healing.* This theory holds that chronic pain can be ignored

---

* Healing may occur on a biochemical level in six to eight weeks, but soft tissue often shortens as it heals, making muscles, tendons, and ligaments tighten, and leaving joints in sub-optimal positions. This "hypo-mobility" needs to be addressed by physical therapists, osteopaths, or chiropractors for health to recur. Often, muscles need to be strengthened as well. The body does some healing by itself, but needs external help with other healing processes.

because it is simply an abnormal firing by the nervous system, and not indicative of new or on-going tissue damage. Of course, many types of chronic pain do involve new or on-going tissue damage, so the theory doesn't apply to them. This theory is sometimes used, however, to try to bully patients into increasing function regardless of pain increases. Some healthcare professionals tell these patients that there's no reason that they shouldn't be functioning at full capacity. The patient is made to feel weak or ashamed, and often responds to this pressure by attempting to do activities that are actually harmful to the patient. In reality, the patient must choose between self-protection and compliance with the healthcare professional's instructions.

Healthcare professionals are supposed to be the patient's advocates, but in this situation they can become adversaries.

In cases where workman's comp, or short- or long-term disability insurance is involved, this situation is compounded. The people evaluating the claims for workman's comp or disability insurance look to the healthcare practitioner, hoping for an indication that the patient should return to work. The health insurance companies hope for the patient to be recovered with as few treatments as possible. These outside factors exert enormous pressures on the patient to be well, but if they can't fully recover, the pressure remains on both the patient and the healthcare practitioner to report that recovery is taking place. People with serious chronic pain problems simply don't fit into this money-driven model. They're seen as problems who stubbornly refuse to get well, and they may be blamed for their own illness.

The pressure increases even further if patients are declared ready to return to work, but in reality are not ready. Literally, their livelihoods are at stake, as the patients cannot receive payments from disability insurance or workman's comp, but also cannot work. If they are unable to return to work within a period of time, they stand to lose both salary and health insurance.

When doctors see patients with different pain levels but similar findings on diagnostic tests, they tend to distrust the patients reporting the most pain. They want to put patients into the same pigeonhole, even though there is a wide variation in individuals. The patient who returns to full function is held up as the model, and the patient who can't function or who has limitations is labeled a failure.

Recent research has shown that individuals vary from one another in pain perception. In 2006, Georgia State University's Professor Anne Murphy reported that men and women feel their pain differently. For example, morphine "works quite differently in the spinal cords of males and females." In fact, "women typically require twice the dosage of morphine to achieve the same degree of pain relief.[1]" This is quite counter-intuitive, because the assumption is usually made that men require higher doses because of their greater body weight. This makes women vulnerable to being under-treated for their pain.

And finally, because chronic pain is difficult to cure, some health care professionals find their egos threatened by it. It's easier to blame the patient than to admit that there are limits to what modern medicine—or health care professionals personally—can achieve.

---

[1] *Research in Gender and Brain Suggests Differences at Cell Level.*, 17 Oct. 2006 <http://www.sfn.org/index.cfm?pagename=news_101706b>

To cope with this bizarre reality, we either needed to laugh or cry. So we did a little of each.

Our humor and our ability to vent emotion got us through many moments of frustration. We decided that to reflect the ironic atmosphere, we would invent "misfortune cookies":

- Things may be going well for you today, but something bad can still happen.

- You have a lot of friends, but they're all talking about you behind your back.

- Your confidence in yourself is an asset; too bad it's misplaced!

- You will have a great success later this year: post-mortem.

- You have the warm feeling that people like you—they're just pretending.

And our personal favorite:

- No matter how bad things may seem, they can always get worse.

Don't ask me why, but we also found relief in coloring books. Maybe it was the simplicity of staying within the lines, or the security of having control over something, but color we did—Sesame Street characters, which we taped up on the walls of our hotel room when we were done. Big Bird, Bert and Ernie, Grover, and Elmo all grinned at us from the walls. You can probably imagine our embarrassment when a maintenance man had to enter our room to service the bathroom. He glanced around and took note of the fact that we didn't have any children staying with us. We laughed hard about that after he left.

We laughed and we cried, but deep inside my soul I knew I needed to come to some acceptance of the pain in my life not being removed. How could I reach acceptance and some degree of peace with this daily and disabling pain? And what about the trauma which had been added by the physicians whose exams had caused additional damage? What could I do to cope with their disrespect and abuse, when all I had been doing was asking for help?

Suing doctors wasn't an option. We were all too aware by this time that diagnostic tests weren't showing the problem. How do you file a lawsuit when you can't document the damage? Pain alone isn't really measurable. So how could I cope?

I looked to the Bible for a spiritual example and found one in the New Testament, in Paul's letter to the Corinthians. Paul wrote:

> There was given me a thorn in the flesh...to torment me. Three times I pleaded with the Lord to take it away from me. But He said to me, "My grace is sufficient for you, for my power is made perfect in weakness" (2 Corinthians 12:7–9).

Scholars don't really know what Paul's "thorn in the flesh" was, but he described it as torment. It sounded like Paul's situation was enough like mine to be relevant. If Paul was able to accept weakness and a "thorn in his flesh" so that God's power could be made perfect in his life, maybe I could learn to look at it that way, too. What did it mean that God's power could be made perfect in my weakness? I think it had to do with God working on my character while I suffered; to help me learn to forgive, to let go of bitterness and resentment. If I could do that, it would only be with God's power. It wasn't my natural response at all.

There was also Romans 12:12; "Be joyful in hope, patient in affliction, faithful in prayer." It was that "patient in affliction" phrase that caught my attention. The Greek word for patient is hupomeno {hoop-om-en'-o}. It means to remain, not to flee, to persevere under misfortune and trial. It implies holding fast to faith in Christ when enduring something difficult; to bear up bravely and calmly when ill-treated. I wanted to persevere; I wanted to have strength for the long haul—but I knew I couldn't muster up this power on my own. I guess that's where the "be faithful in prayer" part came in...if I asked God to help me be "patient in affliction," He would give me the ability to do something impossible for me to do on my own.

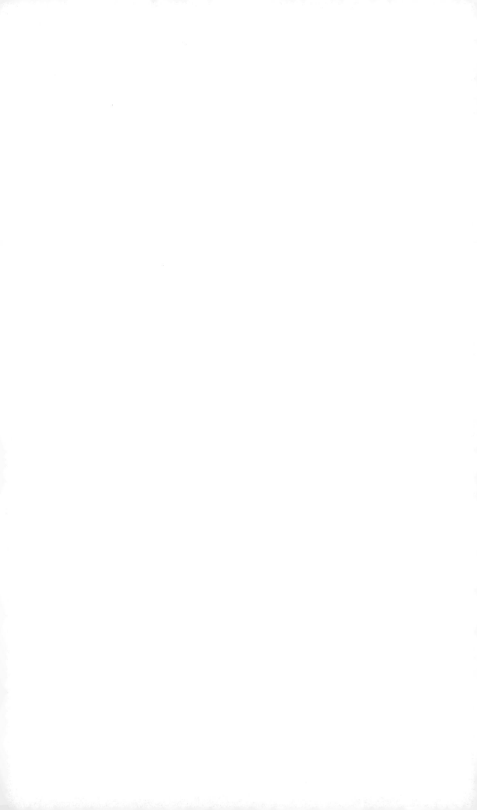

CHAPTER THREE

Adjusting to My Horizontal Life: Finding Ways to Thrive!

Healing Service: God's People Pray

After leaving the pain clinic, my church held a prayer service for me. Our pastor, Ron Zehnder, had called and suggested this idea to us, and we agreed to it. I read a book called *Healing* by Francis MacNutt[1] to prepare for this. I knew enough about the folks in our church to realize that some people were going to want to ask God to heal me miraculously. I was trying to learn more about miraculous healing as experienced by many people in the New Testament as well as in modern times. Apparently, Francis MacNutt was a man who'd seen many—although not all—people healed miraculously by God after he'd prayed for them. Francis McNutt dispelled the myth that the sick person must have faith to be healed, pointing out

---

[1] MacNutt, Francis: "*Healing.*" Creation House, Altamonda Springs, FLA, 1988.

that some individuals in the New Testament were healed even though they didn't know who Jesus was. So it followed that it wasn't neccessarily a lack of faith on my part which kept me from experiencing healing.

At the same time, I had to admit that I wasn't very comfortable with asking for a miracle; I much preferred that God use the avenue of doctors and physical therapists to heal me. However, the medical system really hadn't been able to do much to help us. Maybe God was asking me to step out of my comfort zone. I tried to prepare by thinking about simply being open to healing, in whatever way God wanted to give it. I tried not to insist on being in control of the process, but to be ready to accept God's ways, whatever they were. I wanted to put myself and my future into God's hands; to relinquish control to Him, to His will for my life.

The evening of the prayer service came. Seventy people showed up on a Sunday night to pray for healing and direction in seeking new treatments for my pain. The fact that people would spend an evening praying for me in a spirit of love and concern was very encouraging and humbling. There was a great variety of styles of prayer: some folks, like my pastor, read a verse from the Bible and then said a prayer out loud. Some wanted to anoint me with oil, according to James 5:14–15 :

Is anyone of you sick? He should call the elders of the church to pray over him and anoint him with oil in the name of the Lord. And the prayer offered in faith will make the sick person well; the Lord will raise him up. If he has sinned, he will be forgiven.

This was done by dipping two fingers in oil and using them to make the sign of the cross on my forehead.

Some people wanted to lay hands on me according to Acts 28:8, in which Paul placed his hands on a man and healed him after a time of prayer. I asked them not to touch my back directly. As people placed their hands on me, the sensation of firm pressure on my shoulders, arms, and legs was comforting. Other people prayed quietly in small groupings, or just by themselves. Some asked God for miraculous healing, others asked for help from the medical system, still others for strength to cope with pain now. One prayer stuck out for me, when someone prayed that I would be able to once again run along a beach! Many people prayed that I would simply be able to do normal things again, like sitting and standing for longer periods of time. Others asked that God respond in whatever way He knew was best.

One group wanted me to give them feedback as to whether or not I was experiencing pain relief right then and there. I wasn't. A couple of people wanted to see whether one of my legs was longer than the other, and if so, to "grow" the other one through prayer! As a physical therapist, I knew that leg length can seem to be changed by the positioning of the pelvis, so I didn't give this much credence. One woman actually told me that I should go through my house to see whether there might be any "occult" items, like Ouija boards, which might be blocking the effectiveness of the prayers. That suggestion I quickly dismissed. We discovered that there are very different expectations and approaches that can emerge at a prayer gathering. One man assured me that I had been healed during the prayer time, but unfortunately he was wrong. It's important to try to discern which messages are helpful.

Parts of this experience were a little strange, yet it was very moving to see that many people cared about us and wanted to seek God's help for us. Our friends from church weren't giving up yet, and neither were we.

Two benefits seemed to come out of this prayer service: first, I felt a sense of being spiritually strengthened and supported by God's people. I knew Jesus would help me to face both the situation in which I found myself then and whatever might come next. I felt reassured that God loved me and that He cared deeply about what happened to me. Second, I learned an important piece of information the very next day: coincidence, or divine timing?

The Institute for Low Back Care

On Monday my parents, who live in Iowa, called us. They had been very concerned about the devastating changes in my life which pain had caused. The thousand miles that separated us prevented us from seeing each other as much as we wanted to, especially since travel had become so difficult for me. On their part, they wished they lived closer so that they could help more. They told us about a clinic they'd heard of in Minneapolis which specialized in treating back problems: The Institute for Low Back Care[*]. A clinic that was dedicated to diagnosing and treating spine problems sounded hopeful. If my back problems were unusual, it might take a physician specializing in the spine to figure out what was wrong. My condition was so atypical that I would be happy if

---

[*] The Institute for Low Back Care, currently The Institute for Low Back and Neck Care: ilbnc.com

somebody could even tell me what the problem was. We knew it was degenerative disc disease, but not the typical form. An accurate diagnosis had eluded us so far, and a diagnosis would be the first step to further help. Since Andy's summer vacation from teaching was approaching again, we made an appointment and flew from Detroit to Minneapolis.

Flying was a real nightmare: nothing was accommodated for me. I was told that if I wanted to lie down on the airplane, I would have to pay for four first-class tickets, allowing the airline to remove the seats and bolt down a stretcher. There was no way we could afford that! Since the Americans with Disabilities Act had been passed in the 1990s, there was a lot of talk about accommodating people with disabilities, but it didn't help me. The narrow definition of "disability" which allows for people in wheelchairs to be accommodated didn't include my disability. So I had to lie down at the airport gate until we boarded our plane, sit twenty minutes for take-off, stand for an hour and a half near the flight attendants in the front of the plane (standing being less painful than sitting), sit again twenty minutes for landing, and lie down in the taxi to our hotel. That wiped me out for the rest of the day, and the next day had to be a rest day in our hotel room because of the resultant pain.

My appointment was with Dr. Charles Burton, a surgeon who was well respected in his field, and who specialized in state-of-the-art spinal surgery. After examining me, he ordered an MRI, which showed that my discs were still bulging but not ruptured. I had a selective nerve root block that numbed the sensation from the L5 nerve root. It showed my leg pain was coming from a nerve injury.

Then Dr. Burton ordered a new test I had never had before:

the discogram. Basically a long needle is inserted through layers of muscle in the low back and deep into the disc itself, where dark fluid is injected. A fluoroscopy monitor, like a live x-ray, shows the patient's back and where the fluid goes after being injected. In a healthy disc, the fluid stays in the center of the disc and looks like a dark oval on the fluoroscopy monitor. In two of my discs, the fluid did not stay contained in the center of the disc, but it spread out through large tears in the back of the discs and I experienced excruciating pain.

The discogram is one of the most hellishly painful medical tests known to mankind. Patients are not sedated or anaesthetized during a discogram because they must describe the pain they are feeling to the physician. As I lay on that table in a cold procedure room with three long needles deep inside my back, the doctor injected fluid into my discs, one by one. The disc that was normal just felt like pressure. The two degenerated discs, however, felt like white-hot coals. The agony was so wrenching that I couldn't even speak when the physician performing the test asked me some questions. I had nodded my head slightly to his questions, but he wanted to hear my answers, so I choked them out. "Yes, this test reproduces my usual pain." "Yes, it hurts intensely." "Yes, at that level, too."

With tears streaming down my face, I focused on a single thought: "If this test can finally diagnose my pain, it'll be worth it." The fluoroscopy showed the damaged discs clearly, and the CAT scan done immediately afterward confirmed what the fluoroscopy had shown. My discs had not ruptured and pushed backward in the typical way; they had torn internally, completely through the outer rings. The tears cause a very painful inflammatory cycle with throbbing pain, like a thumb being hit by a hammer. The two lowest discs were very degenerated. Finally we had a diagnostic test that could explain my severe pain!

Dr. Burton sent us back to Michigan with a traction tilt table. I was to strap on a vest and hang suspended from a bar on the tilted platform for thirty minutes, three times per day over the next four months. Unfortunately, this provided little relief or increase in function. Dr. Burton also used radio frequency current to "burn" out small nerve endings to the facet joints that guide movement in my spine — this also was not helpful. To his credit, though, he wanted to exhaust all conservative options before considering surgery.

In November 1992 I returned to Minneapolis for a double fusion surgery under Dr. Burton's care. I had never had a surgery before, and I went into it with great hopes and optimism. This surgeon had, after all, been the one who finally figured out what the problem was. In the seven-hour surgery, Dr. Burton removed the damaged discs and fused the vertebra above to the vertebra below (or the sacrum) at each level. At that time the fusion cages were new. They were like large, hollow screws which he placed between my bones. They had been developed in response to failures that occurred when only bone was placed between vertebrae to create a fusion. Having the hollow metal cage to guide the bone growth made them less likely than bone grafts alone to fail to fuse.

So I received two titanium fusion cages at L5-S1 but a femoral bone graft[*] at L4-5 since anatomically there wasn't enough width at that level for the cages. Interestingly enough, the cages were successful as expected, but the bone graft

---

[*] a cross-section of a femur, or leg-bone, from a cadaver

failed to fuse. I had to wear a huge magnetic belt ten hours a day for six months to stimulate bone growth. Eventually that was successful. Once the surgical pain healed, I was amazed to find that for the first time in 2 ½ years, my disc pain was gone! I still had some back and leg pain from nerve injury, but the deep, severe, midline pain from the damaged discs was behind me. Hurray! We were ecstatic to share this news with friends and family. My parents were especially heartened by this news, as my dad had several back surgeries himself.

Dr. Burton informed us that the disc tissue he removed was supposed to be the consistency of crab meat; my disc tissue was the consistency of mucous. What a relief that there was a true physical explanation to my disabling pain. This additional physical evidence was very validating for me, especially after the pain clinic's suggestion that my personality had been at fault! It cemented my belief that I should trust my body and listen to my body. The pain messages had indicated tissue damage—and accurately. My body's pain signals were reliable even in the absence of diagnostic tests results. Sometimes the right diagnostic tests just haven't been invented yet!

We made seven trips back and forth to Minneapolis in all. It was a hopeful time for us, and we were very grateful to Dr. Burton. I began a walking program and progressed to walking up to two miles a day! I still couldn't sit long because of the leg pain, but during this time I was able to go to the university to study German for six semesters. Andy was a German teacher, and I wanted to understand the German language, culture, and politics better. Throughout Andy's career, we would be hosting visiting teachers from Germany and their students, and I would be able to relate to them more easily. I also completed a children's literature writing course through the mail. Even though writing was hard work, I enjoyed being mentally productive. My life seemed as if it were moving toward something again, rather than stagnating. Since sitting was still difficult, Andy worked hard to adapt a computer so I could use it lying down, allowing me to do some volunteer word processing and desktop publishing for a local mission organization. I could be on the computer for a couple of hours per day. I felt more productive and optimistic and had more concrete goals than I'd been able to set for myself in several years.

My Outcome

The fusion surgery had addressed the first component of my problem: discogenic pain. There was, however, a second component: neurogenic pain, or pain coming from injured nerves. Could we find treatments helpful for the nerve injury and leg pain?

My physical therapist, Pam Perkins, attended a continuing education class on nerve root injury. She consulted with the presenter, David S. Butler[2], on my case. He said disc bulging had caused the initial nerve damage. My bending forward in the shower, way back in 1990 when my disc had been bulging, had aggravated that. After that, aggressive physician exams, specifically the straight leg raises performed over and over again, had caused further nerve injury. Mr. Butler's impression was that I had an overstretch injury to the whole lumbosacral nerve plexus. This is a group of nerves that go from the spine to the leg and include the large sciatic nerve.

---

[2] Butler, David S., "Mobilisation of the Nervous System," Churchill Livingston, 1991.

Nerves have two components: the fibers which carry the electrical signals and the connective tissue surrounding those fibers. In my case, the connective tissue had been damaged. Every time the straight leg raise was repeated, the re-stretching would cause what Mr. Butler termed "hospital-level pain," or pain which is too severe to manage at home. Mr. Butler cautioned that was never to be done again with me. The main problem was with the L5 nerve root on the right side, which agreed with Dr. Burton's finding of nerve root compression in surgery. Dr. Burton had decompressed the nerve root, but permanent damage had already occurred. There really wasn't any treatment for this. The best we could do was to manage the symptoms. When Pam relayed this news to me, it depressed me, because I knew that this would mean life-long limitations. Until now, I had hoped for a return to more-or-less normal function. Andy and I were both sad; we realized that our lives were taking a different path than we would have ever chosen.

I was unable to return to working as a physical therapist because of the permanent nerve damage. My boss reluctantly removed my name and my job title from the board in the entryway of the clinic. My two-year long-term disability policy came to an end. The company decided I was not "permanently and totally disabled," so the benefits were terminated. Social Security made a similar determination. Andy and I thought those decisions were unjust, and we considered hiring an attorney to represent me in court. However, more doctor exams would be required. Every time I was examined, especially with the straight leg raise test, my leg pain would worsen with such severity that I had to go to the pain clinic to have an epidural steroid injection. It took a month to get an appointment, and three to five days after that for the injection to work. Besides, each time the straight leg raise test was performed it seemed the nerve was stretched and damaged further.

Even though I still was very limited by my condition, we made the decision not to pursue any legal avenues because of the required physician exams. Once again, there weren't clear diagnostic tests that showed the nerve damage. The existing diagnostic tests measured damage to the electrical signal, not the connective tissue. Legally I would have a weak case. I don't know what would have happened if Mr. Butler, or someone like him, had been called as an expert witness. We never found out. We just weren't going to allow one more doctor to examine me and to try to force the straight leg raise test on me. This decision made things harder for us financially, but we were convinced that protecting my body was more important.

I tried acupuncture for six months, but it didn't alter my symptoms. My neurologist and osteopath, Dr. Elkiss, did cranio-sacral therapy, which helped somewhat. By pushing and pulling on the skin over my skull, he was able to indirectly help my back. The cranium, or skull, is connected to the spine and sacrum. Mild stretches can be applied through the dura mater, the tough layer of connective tissue overlying the brain and spinal cord. Dr. Elkiss recommended eastern herb tinctures, which I took but found it difficult to assess their effects.

By this time I had switched to another pain clinic in our area. A psychologist there worked with me to learn biofeedback, a method of learning deep muscle relaxation. He also taught me visualization: "Picture your pain as an island of discomfort in a sea of relaxation." The deep relaxation is something I began to use every day and it could "reset" my pain by reducing it a couple of points. Pain can be rated on a scale from 1-10, with 1 being very little pain and ten being excruciating. With deep relaxation and visualization I could reduce the pain from a six to a four or five, but only temporarily.

For exercise* I found swimming or doing water exercises to be the best, because the buoyancy of the water unloaded my spine. I could do motions in the water, like jogging, which my back would have never tolerated on land. I began exercising twenty minutes in the water, three times a week, and added ten minutes of careful stretching at the end.

My results with walking varied more. Some days it was helpful to walk; other days walking severely aggravated my pain. I decided that I would like to live on the moon, where gravity would be less of a problem. Barring that, perhaps we should live under water, since it seemed to be my best friend. We invested in a Jacuzzi for our backyard deck, and every evening I spent half an hour sitting —yes, sitting—in the 105 degree water as the jets massaged my aching, sore muscles, which were often in spasm.

I was prescribed a TENS unit, which stands for Transcutaneous Electrical Nerve Stimulation. It was a portable, battery-operated unit with wires connecting it to flat, flexible square electrodes. The electrodes could be placed on the skin over my back and leg, where I felt the tight, cramping pain. When I turned the TENS unit on, it felt like a tingling or a buzzing under the electrodes. This muted the sensation of

---

* A good guideline for exercise is that your pain may increase afterward because the tissue has been stressed somewhat. By the next day, however, the pain should be back to normal levels. If it isn't, you may have done too much exercise or the wrong type of exercise for your condition.

pain somewhat.

I tried several back braces. The rigid plastic ones, heavy and unyielding, cinched so tight that they bothered my ribs and I could hardly eat anything. Wearing them felt like living in a body cast. I preferred a back support made out of cloth, elastic and Velcro, which supported me a little when I was vertical, but which wasn't so unyielding.

Regarding pain medications, my neurologist prescribed 800 mg. Ibuprofen tablets and Vicodin, an opiate or narcotic. For years I took the Ibuprofen around the clock, and when my pain got to a five or higher on a scale from one to ten, I'd take the Vicodin in addition. It wouldn't eliminate the pain, but it could reduce it to tolerable levels if I also lay down. Pain medications alone were not enough. I also had to exercise in the pool, use the TENS unit, and lie down frequently throughout the day to manage the pain.

Pain Flares: Testing My Survival Skills

Pain flares brought even greater challenges. When my pain would flare and worsen dramatically, I had to resume full bed rest for several days, only getting up to go to the bathroom. My pain felt like it was screaming at me. Gradually I could begin some gentle movements in a pool or jacuzzi. I imagined the function that was returning as a seedling emerging from soil. If I added function too quickly, the seedling would be ripped from the ground. It had to be protected and cared for until its roots were better established. If I was very patient and very careful, over a few days I could add a few more minutes of vertical time each day. The seedling of function would become stronger. As more days passed, my function would return to "my normal" levels, having two to four hours out of bed per day. The pain would recede to "my normal" level of pain, about a four or five on a scale from one to ten. But any error or misjudgment in this process would eradicate the progress and send me back to full bed rest again. If I did too much, I would just set myself back.

It was truly challenging to live so carefully and to have so little room for error. But thinking about my function as a fragile plant helped me to be gentle with myself. It helped to have an example from nature—a seedling—with which I could compare my situation.

From a physical therapy point of view, when my pain flared it was because the tissue in my back was irritated and inflamed. It is well-established that inflammation causes chemical pain which sets off small nerve endings, transmitting the pain message up the spinal cord and to the brain. Involuntary muscle guarding and spasms result. Four phases of recovery followed. Phase one was rest and applying ice. Phase two was gentle movements to minimize swelling and to improve motion. Heat and massage also helped reduce muscle spasms. Phase three was minimal exercise and stretching. Phase four was moderate exercise to regain or increase strength, followed by stretching to improve flexibility. These phases would have to be implemented again every time I had a pain flare.

Taking care of my back took a great deal of time and effort. When you counted the doctor visits, physical therapy appointments, exercise time, and rest time, not to mention the pain flares, it was like having a full-time job.

It's hard to believe that pain from a nerve plexus injury can be so disabling. How can pain in a small region of the body control the rest of that body? I can't fully explain it; I

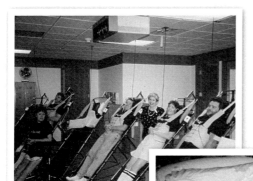

Above: The Institute for Low Back Care.

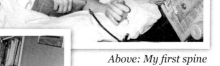

Above: My first spine surgery.

Above: Adapting the computer.

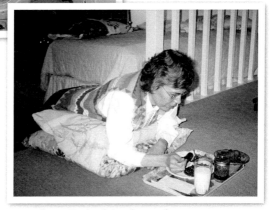

Above: Eating lying forward over a step.

only know what the experience has been like for me. Before I had this kind of pain, I would never have understood it. I am not a frail person, and I've been told that I have an excellent pain tolerance. All I can say is that this condition changed my life and forced me into a life of lying down twenty-two hours a day. With this condition, I considered myself disabled. I felt trapped.

It's also difficult to communicate the level of loss which came with my condition or disability. While disabled people in wheelchairs can travel and go places, my disability largely prevented me from travel. I missed my parents' fiftieth wedding anniversary celebration, which all of my siblings were able to attend. I was unable to travel to attend my sister Judy's wedding. Family reunions were sometimes scheduled where I live, other times not—and I had to be excluded from those. There was significant, real emotional pain which accompanied the physical pain. I seem to miss out on the celebration events of life: weddings, birthday parties, graduations, etc. Not being able to attend the significant events of the people I love is one of my deepest wounds.

So there was the physical situation, but also an emotional and social side to these difficult circumstances.

Swimming Pool

The swimming pool in the city recreation building is a great equalizer, a rare shared environment for the able and disabled, young and old, the weak and the strong. Some labels are cast off in the act of putting on a swimsuit: "white collar professional", "blue collar laborer," "stay at home mom," "stylish/trendy," and "slacker;" while other labels remain:

"woman with scoliosis," "man with multiple sclerosis," "person in a wheelchair," and "young woman with an amputation". My label, "horizontal woman," can be cast off temporarily, because my stay is so brief. I can look normal for a short while. It is therapy to my soul to see so many people with various limitations, because I don't feel so alone ... although to them I'm sure I appear normal for the short time that they see me.

A few people with disabilities there have become friends over the years. There's John, who broke his neck in a car accident, which paralyzed him and killed his fiancée. He comes to float in a vest and move his arms in the water, helping to prevent pressure sores from sitting in his wheelchair so much. Now, John doesn't come any more, because it takes him and his assistant two hours just to get him up in the morning, and another two hours to get through the pool and locker room. Then there's James, who's so very thin and also needs a wheelchair because he has multiple sclerosis. He walks sideways down the ramp into the water with difficulty, clinging to the railing, because his legs have trouble obeying his brain's commands with much strength or coordination. James is patient, ever so patient, "swimming" back and forth wearing a foam vest, but mostly pushing water around with his arms as his legs dangle. He moved to San Diego to be in a better climate for his MS.

There's Chris who is very short due to a serious congenital bone condition. She has endured multiple bone fractures—over twenty different times in her lifetime. She walks with crutches and is incredibly courageous to come out and swim laps, when any fall could mean another fracture. There's also the man who takes baby steps and shuffles across the room ever so slowly, although his steps are very rapid. Does he have

Parkinson's disease? Then there's the young woman with only one arm and some type of mental impairment. She is shy and tentative in the water. The older women exercise together in a class to ease arthritic pain, their limps disappearing for an hour and only re-appearing when they climb out of the water. These are all the quiet heroes, going about their days facing obstacles most others are spared, and rarely being recognized for it.

Mixed throughout are the healthy and the strong, muscular and toned. They swim their hundreds of laps, do their flip-turns and reach their target heart rates. They easily push themselves out of the water when they're through, not bothering to use the ladder. As they walk past the people with disabilities, I think, "This is their chance to realize their incredible fortune at being healthy and strong." And maybe that thought crosses some of their minds. But perhaps they don't see the disabled; perhaps subconsciously they believe they are entitled to health, and that others are entitled to disability. I know I used to take my strength and ability for granted. Or maybe it's just too frightening to contemplate: the vulnerability of the human condition, how each of us is just one accident or diagnosis away from disability.

So I continue to strike up conversations with people in both situations—the weak and the strong—and I tell them my story briefly, so they understand that some disabilities are invisible. And I ask the folks who struggle through life where they get their strength—ironically, it takes internal strength to be externally weak—and how they deal with limits. Sometimes I feel guilty that their disabilities are more profound than mine. Ah, but pain is such a difficult thing to measure, and I may look fine, but every lap I swim is through thicker waters in a sea of pain. I make small talk with anyone who is willing, because the pool is the only place I go three times a week. It's the only place I drive myself—twelve minutes each way—and an important connection to the outside world for me.

Support Group

For several years I led a support group for women with chronic pain in my home. We had all responded to a newspaper ad for women with chronic pain. After being in a fee-for-service therapy group for eight weeks, we chose to continue meeting on our own. We used resources from several national[3] groups to pick our topics for meetings. Mostly, though, we benefited from sharing our personal stories with each other and giving and receiving support. It was a relief to be with this small group of women who also understood life with varying levels of chronic pain.

Mary: Ever since I fell on ice last winter and felt something tear, I have back pain every day. I can still function at a pretty high level, enough to work as an engineer. But after work, my life is lying down and dealing with pain.

Katie: I know what you mean. I can work part-time, but feel like I have no life outside of that. Doctor's appointments, physical therapy—that's all I do.

Joanna: You two can still work. Must be nice. I had to retire from nursing in my forties because my pain was so bad. I just couldn't help lift the patients any more or help them

---

[3] The American Chronic Pain Association, The National Chronic Pain Outreach Association, and Rest Ministries.

transfer in and out of bed.

Agnes: I'm sad for all you younger women. At least my pain didn't start until I was in my sixties. I had a normal life until then.

Roxanne: To be honest, I envy all of you. Mine started at twenty-seven, and I haven't been able to work since, or function much at all. But at least you understand how hard it is to have pain every day.

Mary: Oh, I know, it's so invisible; other people don't think there's really anything wrong with you. But it's so very real. And pain makes it hard to make plans. Richard wants me to go away for the weekend. If I'm having a good day, that might be fun. But if I'm having a bad day, it will be agony. All I can think about is wanting to stay home so I don't risk hurting so much.

Joanna: And even if you do stay home, it's not like you can accomplish much. I have to pace myself to do any gardening at all. Twenty minutes is about my limit, and I used to spend hours.

Agnes: I'm a widow, and it got so hard to do things in the yard, I moved to a condo.

Katie: I hate having to ask my husband to do everything I can't do. I mean, I'm glad he's there to help me, but I just feel so useless sometimes, like a burden.

Roxanne: That sounds familiar. I feel so helpless and powerless lying down when there are dirty dishes to wash, a lawn to mow, laundry to be done … and even though I do the little that I can do, so much of it falls on Andy. It's not fair to him.

Agnes: But it's not like you chose pain just to get out of work. You would have never chosen this lifestyle.

Roxanne: Definitely not! I would give almost anything to be healthy and strong again. I'd even be thrilled to clean a toilet, if it didn't hurt me so much.

Joanna: What do we do with our feelings of guilt, that we can't do as much as we want to do; that our families end up doing more than their fair share?

Mary: It just makes me want to disappear sometimes, to escape into something, and not deal with my feelings about it.

Katie: I guess I try to thank Shannon whenever he does things around the house. I know it isn't much, but I try to let him know that I appreciate his efforts.

Roxanne: There are a few things I can do lying down that help Andy, like writing a grocery list, keeping track of our budget, or doing our taxes. But Andy definitely does more.

Mary: Making any kind of a contribution helps. I just feel better about myself.

Katie: I pay our bills and do some of the cooking.

Agnes: There's not much at all that I can do. I guess I just try to be nice to other people, like my cleaning lady. I figure she doesn't need to hear about all my problems.

Joanna: And then your cleaning lady can see that you're trying to be friendly despite your pain—that's good. Just having a good attitude can be hard work for us.

Roxanne: Then am I doing the wrong thing by telling Andy how depressed I get? For me, the feelings have to be expressed sometimes, when I can't hold them in any longer. I might tell him that I'm angry or frustrated or whatever.

Mary: Is that the only way you relate to him?

Roxanne: Oh, no. He usually listens to me and says something supportive, and then after a while I can move on and talk about other things.

Katie: That sounds healthy to me. With me and Shannon, he says he'd rather have me tell him what's bugging me instead of just being irritable. Even though he can't do anything to fix my pain.

Joanna: Yeah, that's hard for guys. They want to be able to fix things. Don gets very frustrated that in spite of all my doctor's visits and surgeries, I'm still in pain. That drives him crazy.

Agnes: I remember that sometimes I just wanted my husband to empathize. But it's hard on husbands, too, seeing us in pain, and feeling so powerless to help us.

Roxanne: The best thing Andy says to me is that if he had the pain I have, he'd feel just as depressed or angry or desperate as I do.

Mary: He says that?

Roxanne: He really does. He lets me be real about my feelings, and he tries to empathize. But he stops me if I start to project my pain into the future. Like if I tell him, "This will never get any better" or "I can't imagine living like this the rest of my life." It doesn't help me, and it might not be true anyway.

Katie: That's great, Roxanne, Andy is such a natural at this role.

Roxanne: Just remember, he had to grow into it. Nobody sat him down when we got married and taught him how to be supportive or encouraging. He just learned it by trying things out. But he was open to learning, and I'm very grateful to him for that.

Mary: So, if my husband doesn't know how to support me, how do I get him to start?

Agnes: Well, actually, you might consider telling him what could help you at times like that. If he has an idea what to say, he might be willing to try it.

Katie: You'd have to be subtle, because men don't like to be told what to do.

Joanna: Don would probably be okay with hearing a suggestion, especially if he knew it could help calm me down when I'm upset.

Mary: Oh, heck, even if our husbands don't always get it, we have each other, right? You guys can call me anytime you need to talk.

Agnes: That goes for me, too. You can call me any time.

Joanna: What would we do without girlfriends?

Roxanne: Oh! I can't imagine!

Katie: I need my girlfriends as much as I need oxygen!

After three years, the support group disbanded. Katie and Mary recovered; Katie went on to have a baby and open her own business; Mary's life returned to normal. Agnes' pain worsened so she couldn't attend meetings, and Joanna began traveling a lot with her husband. It is possible that sharing some of my experience as a longer-term person with pain and my knowledge as a physical therapist helped some of them find their healing paths. I felt like I had at least made a contribution.

As for me, my pain was still a big factor in my life. I missed the support group but had probably learned as much as I was going to learn from these particular women. I remember thinking, though, that pain conditions were a temporary problem for many people while I seemed to get the permanent life sentence, and how unfair that was. The fact that Agnes didn't get relief from her pain, though, reminded me that I wasn't alone. It seemed that the other support group members visited the land of pain and limitations, but Agnes and I were permanent residents there.

A Loyal, Long-Term Physician

Dr. Mitch Elkiss has been my long-term doctor since 1991. We drive an hour one-way every two months to see him. On the way, we pass other health systems, hospitals, and doctor's offices because he is a rare find. Dr. Elkiss is both a neurologist and an osteopath. His case load includes patients with neurological conditions such as multiple sclerosis, epilepsy, neuropathy, migraines, and chronic neck or back pain. Many of his patients have long-term conditions, which must be managed over the years rather than cured.

I have found Dr. Elkiss to be very knowledgeable in his field, to have excellent skills both as a neurologist and an osteopath, and to be willing to treat me over a long period of time: many years! It is rare to find a physician who is as patient as he is, and as optimistic in looking for small gains. His criteria for success, I believe, are individualized to each patient. Instead of having only one measure of success, such as returning to work or returning to full function, he measures success in realistic ways. His goal is to maximize each patient's potential, but to accept that patients have limitations after illness or injury. The management of these conditions is a valid goal, even if there is minimal improvement. More significantly, his treatments keep many patients from losing ground.

It is also wonderful to have one doctor to whom to turn for advice on prescriptions, for referrals, and with whom to discuss new treatment options being considered. The stability of having one doctor who sticks by you is priceless, especially when your medical file is inches thick, and he is willing to oversee your case and try to make sense of it all.

In turn, I try to be a respectful, compliant patient. There have been times when I've disagreed with doctors, but usually not Dr. Elkiss. His assessments are right-on. I appreciate the fact that he allows me to be part of the decision-making process, and he is not threatened by the fact that I'm an informed patient. Over the years he has become a cherished physician and partner in my healthcare.

Dr. Elkiss prescribed a subtherapeutic dose of an antidepressant medication for its ability to raise my pain threshold, making me somewhat less perceptive to pain. He prescribed Neurontin, an anti-seizure drug that is useful with nerve pain. He offered, at various times, acupuncture, herbal remedies, craniosacral therapy, and osteopathic mobilizations. He has written letters of introduction for me which I've taken to appointments with new surgeons. He's written referrals for me to receive epidural injections at pain clinics. Most of all, though, I cherish his ability to listen combined with excellent problem solving skills and encouragement.

If you can find a doctor like this, consider yourself very fortunate! I would think twice—or three times!—about moving somewhere else and having to start over with a new physician.

Interview with Dr. Elkiss

Q: You are an osteopath, rather than an M.D. Can you explain the difference?

A: I am an Osteopathic physician. The philosophy of Osteopathic medicine includes the idea that the body is self-regulating. This leads the effort of patient care to be focused on enhancing the body's natural ability. It recognizes the inherent medicine chest that the human being possesses. Treatment is directed at optimizing the capacity of the body to produce the proper mix of internal chemistry. Together these offer a respect for the natural intelligence that the human organism possesses. This intelligence surpasses even the knowledge of the physician.

Osteopathic medicine acknowledges the reciprocal relation of structure and function. If structure is impaired, then function will be affected. If function is disturbed, then structure will become altered. It is for these reasons that osteopathic therapeutics are aimed at normalizing function and maximizing the efficient structural relationships of the body's systems. There is an intricate interrelatedness that exists between all body systems. This is part of the dynamic assessment of individuals that is part of the osteopathic evaluation. The interrelatedness extends beyond the individual alone to include their family, their workplace, their community, and their socio-cultural group. This is what is known as holism. The individual is more than the sum of their parts.

Q: How does the osteopathic philosophy influence the way you practice medicine?

A: A particularly important aspect of osteopathic medicine is the use of palpatory diagnosis of the neuro-muscular-skeletal system. This reveals information that is a measure of structural pathology of the somatic system, as well as a reflection of internal disorders. Additionally, this provides an opportunity to manually affect changes in the structural presentation of the individual. This can promote healthy structural and functional relations. The dependence on palpatory diagnosis necessitates the close examination of the patient and the laying on of hands. This fosters a bonding between patient and doctor that is unique.

Q: You also have become skilled in acupuncture and other forms of alternative medicine (newer term "integrative medicine"). How do these types of therapies fit into chronic pain management?

A: Integrative medicine implies the integration of multiple disciplines and modalities in the treatment of patients. In chronic pain management, it is well-accepted that a multi-disciplinary approach is most successful. Having more tools in the toolbox affords a higher probability of having the right tool for the job. In addition, an integrative approach facilitates the incorporation of multiple techniques, as well as multiple practitioners, into the therapeutic team. The goal is to have the patient as captain of that team. It also promotes the open and informed consideration of all potential therapies. Acupuncture in particular can be valuable because it is safe, non-toxic, and relatively easy to perform. It allows an analysis of the problem through an entirely different perspective, which at times can be uniquely beneficial. It has particular value in neuro-musculo-skeletal pain management, but at its highest levels, is designed to act at the preventative level.

Q: Many physicians seem to be uncomfortable with patients who don't get well. What is your philosophy in working with patients with chronic conditions? (Is it a valid goal to maintain function, or must it always be increased?)

A: Some physicians are uncomfortable with patients who

don't get well. I think that is the case when they believe that it is their responsibility to get them well. Then they feel that they have failed, making them feel uncomfortable, and often making them seek a distance from those patients. On the other hand, I believe that it is the patient's job to make their own self well. The physician is there to help inform, instruct, guide, facilitate, and treat the patient, to help create a circumstance that maximizes the patient's potential for healing and wellness. A valid goal is any goal that seeks to optimize the functions and quality of a person's life. Moving forward, maintaining function, and even minimizing loss of function can all be valid therapeutic objectives. Forming a partnership between doctor and patient helps to introduce wellness responsibility to the naïve patient and reinforces the goals of therapy to the experienced patient.

Adaptations

As it began to look more and more like I would need to remain a "horizontal woman" to manage my pain, we started putting energy into adapting my life. As a couple, Andy and I were committed to doing whatever we could that would allow me to participate in day-to-day life. Since riding in a car while sitting caused me severe pain, we bought a minivan. Andy removed a bucket seat and bench seat in the back, leaving space for a mattress six feet long by two feet wide on the floor of the van. Next he worked with the University of Michigan Orthotics department. The head of the department, Mr. Mark Taylor, had a disability himself—post polio syndrome—and was sympathetic to my situation. The goal was to fabricate "seat belts" for me to use lying down in our van.

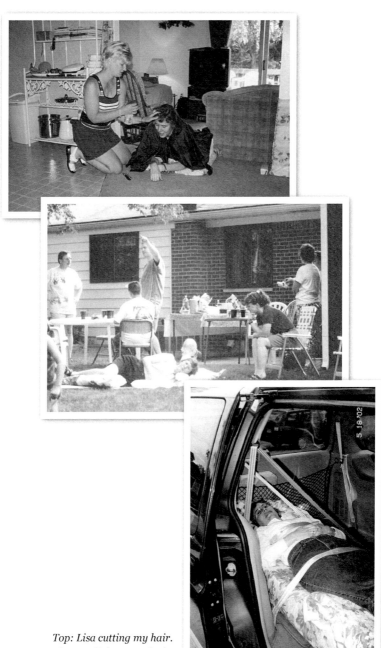

Top: Lisa cutting my hair.
Center: Going to a picnic.
Bottom: Adapting our minivan.

Andy looked at gurneys in ambulances to figure out where the restraints should go, and he constructed samples which the orthotics department converted into actual belts with their industrial-strength sewing machines. One restraining belt went across my rib cage and the second across my legs above my knees. I was still limited in terms of how far I could travel, even lying down, because of the vibration from the road. On a bad day, I was unable to travel at all, but on a good day I could travel in the van two hours, and on a great day, four to five hours. This was a huge improvement over the thirty-minute maximum I could travel sitting up.

Andy also got me a laptop computer which he put on a tilting desk. I could recline backward in a chair about forty-five degrees and use the computer suspended above me. On a good day, I could be in this position for up to an hour-and-a-half before my pain worsened. That adaptation meant I could exchange e-mail, do research on the Internet, and write articles. One year I published a monthly newsletter using this adapted position. The computer served as one avenue to connect me with the outside world.

Imagine not being able to sit in any room of your own home. The furniture would be basically useless! So, a third adaptation Andy made was to put a daybed in every room of our house. It was important for me to be able to change location from room to room and to feel a part of family life or friends' visits wherever they were happening in the house. I needed a bed like some people need a wheel chair, only beds can't roll from room to room.

My fourth adaptation was the result of compassion from a friend. My good friend Lisa usually cuts hair in her own beauty salon in her home. For me, though, she started coming to my house to give me haircuts. On a good day, I sit on a Scandinavian kneeling chair for a quick ten-minute cut. On a worse day, I lie on the floor, and Lisa kneels next to me to cut my hair. Lisa is one of God's gifts in my life.

Our fifth adaptation was for when we went somewhere away from home. We found a camping cot to be useful. Andy would set up the cot, lay a wooden board across the top of it to prevent sagging, and cover the board with a foam mat. This allowed me to lie down above the ground or floor, so I could be seen more easily with less danger of anyone tripping over me or falling onto me. It was also easier to make eye contact with other people and not feel much lower than everyone else.

Of course, adaptations have their limits. When we were invited to see a play at the University of Michigan Power Center, I called the ticket office and asked to speak to a supervisor. I explained my disability and how it was different from the typical categories people imagine when adapting public spaces. I was not a person needing a wheelchair, or visually-impaired, hearing-impaired or mobility-impaired. I simply could not sit and would need to lie down to attend a play. The supervisor listened and thought for a moment. She said that the ticket office would be willing to sell me four tickets usually reserved for wheelchair users. I'd have to bring my own cot, and I would have an excellent view of the back of the seats in front of me, not the stage. So I could pay four times as much as everyone else and not see a thing! Not too surprisingly, I let this wonderful opportunity pass me by.

It frustrated me that society's definitions of disability were so narrow, and that most people really wouldn't even try to accommodate me. It felt like I was being excluded from most public environments which other people take for granted.

People in public spaces are generally required or expected to be vertical. The isolation caused by this fact made this suffering worse.

For the same reason I am unable to go to movie theaters, concerts, sporting events, or restaurants. I can't ride on a train or a bus, and I almost never fly. Can you imagine your life without any of these activities? Only if you can imagine not being able to sit, stand, or walk for more than a few minutes a day.

Our church, however, was aware of our situation and had compassion for me. When they planned a building expansion, they included a special needs room in the blueprints. It would be at the back of the church and have a daybed and recliner in it so someone like me could lie down during church. I would be able to see what was going on through a glass wall and the sound would be brought in through speakers.

What an incredible act of sensitivity and inclusion! When it was finished, I couldn't get over the fact that a public space had been accommodated for me, and I would never have to miss church because of pain. Every time I used the room it seemed like a gift that could be opened again and again. It was a physical, visual reminder that all were welcome and had a place. Gradually other people used it, too, if they had a need. Some used it because they were undergoing chemotherapy and found it difficult to sit upright in a pew. Others had heart or vascular problems for which they needed to elevate their legs. Hopefully this room helped send a message to people in our community that those with disabilities are welcome!

Point System

Many days, my pain dogged me from the moment I got up in the morning. Quite frequently, however, my pain seemed to flare several hours or even a day after I did some activity. This delayed pain made it hard to know when I was "overdoing it." Each morning I would wake up and assess my pain levels. If I had a lot of pain right away, I would force myself to lie down most of the day. On days when I woke up in the morning and felt less pain, I would stand, sit, or walk for fifteen minutes or half an hour at a time. Over the course of a day, this could add up to as many as four hours out of bed. Many days I wouldn't lie down for good until the pain started to worsen. By then it was too late, as the delayed pain would still be increasing several hours later, even though I would have been lying down during that time. This can happen with inflammatory conditions, where swelling occurs several hours after the tissue is stressed or loaded.

It occurred to me that I might be able to keep my pain levels from spiking so much if I did a little bit less of the activity which would provoke the pain. But how much activity was okay with my back, and how would I learn to measure activity? I knew that sitting required more from my back than standing, because that's what I experienced. Disc pressures have actually been measured in a scientific study[4], and sitting

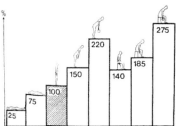

The pressure on the semi-liquid center of the disc changes with position.

[4] "Nachemson's Graphics"

puts twice as much pressure on discs as standing. So I decided to count ten minutes of sitting as two points, but ten minutes of standing would only cost me one point.

I would start by allowing myself five points of function per day on a bad pain day, but ten points of function on a moderate pain day. I thought about all the activities I usually did over the course of a week or month, and assigned each activity a point value. For example, driving sitting upright for ten minutes cost me a point, but I could ride in the passenger seat—reclined—for thirty minutes for that same point. I could get three times the function out of my back by simply being a passenger instead of the driver. Along the same lines, if I lay flat on the mattress in the back of the van, I could ride 45 minutes for one point.

This system of having points to spend each day gave me an unexpected gift: in addition to stabilizing my pain better from day to day, it helped me to focus on the function I had, rather than on the myriad of things I couldn't do. It helped me feel like I had some choice each day about how I would use my points. Using the point system required discipline, much like budgeting money does. But if I could minimize the occurrence of pain spikes—the equivalent of bounced checks—it would be worth it. It was a positive way of looking at—and living with—my back, which didn't feel so much like the enemy.

Clearly, there were activities that were never going to be okay with my back: going bowling or skiing, for example, or even sitting in a theater for two hours to watch a movie. I have had to say goodbye to these things for this life. I have fairly severe limitations, and other people may have moderate or minimal limitations. If you need to manage your activity, or you know someone who does, please see Appendix C to personalize this system for yourself.

Needing Help

Having limitations prevented me from being as self-reliant as I wanted to be. It was awkward to need help from others. I had gone from being one of the "fitter" members of society to being one of the more fragile. Suddenly, I needed to ask a family member or friend to lift a gallon of milk, open a heavy door, give me a ride, or run an errand for me. All my life—for twenty-seven years—I'd been strong, able to help, able to be a caregiver. As a physical therapist, I helped others recover from injuries and surgeries. Now I needed help and care.

It didn't seem right to burden other people with my needs. My dependence, especially when asking for rides, made me feel like I was about twelve years old again. Back in college and graduate school, I had driven myself all around the country without giving it a second thought. The contrast to now was enormous. I had moved my possessions in and out of dorms and apartments, easily lifting furniture and heavy boxes. Now I couldn't even lift a gallon of milk. I was also very self-conscious of the fact that if I went to visit extended family, others would have to do all the physical work of serving a meal or washing the dishes or doing whatever needed to be done. I was especially bothered by this whenever we went to visit my eighty-year-old parents. It was such a role-reversal; I wanted to serve them, but they needed to serve me. Stoic self-reliance had been a large part of my family's German heritage; it was good to work hard, and bad not to. And in my younger years, I certainly had worked hard, toiling in the Iowa farm fields, de-tassling corn for eight-hour days in the summer, for example. But this wasn't laziness; it was disability/inability. Nevertheless, I wrestled with feelings of guilt and uselessness.

It didn't help that western culture views disabled people as noncontributing members of society. They are marginalized and viewed as incapable, unable, and possibly even a burden. In the public sphere, many gains have been made in accommodating people with wheelchairs, especially those who can still use their arms. However, we have a long way to go. Whole groups of people still struggle to find their place in society, to say nothing of trying to find gainful employment. The blind, the deaf, those with head injuries or mental impairments, those with chronic illnesses or chronic pain are often overlooked or pushed aside in favor of the strong and the capable—"normal"—people.

But relying on strength can be a trap. Even people who seem especially strong and successful in society's eyes have vulnerabilities. To be human is to be vulnerable to accidents, illnesses, even to premature death. The able-bodied are just one diagnosis or accident away from being ill or disabled. It can all change in a split second.

One day a friend suggested the concept of interdependence. I didn't want to be dependent upon others; I couldn't be independent any more, but the idea of interdependence is that each person has something to give—and receive—from others. I needed physical help sometimes, but I had things I could give others who helped me: a listening ear, a thoughtful response, or perhaps a prayer spoken for them. Beginning to focus on the needs of others and what I could give to them made it easier to ask for help when I needed something.

The saying goes, "It is more blessed to give than to receive." People have told me it's true. I just need to trust that they're being honest, and that in some mysterious way God gives them a blessing for helping me. It may also be easier to give out of strength than to receive out of weakness, because weakness can make one feel helpless and inadequate. Again, it helped to focus on what I had to give.

Going a level deeper, though, even if I had nothing to give to anyone else, I had to see that I had value simply by being a child of God. Being carefully designed and created by God gives each human being dignity and worth, completely apart from anything they can do. The Bible says that people are created in the image of God and have inherent value. God values and esteems all human life.

God doesn't see our worth as what we do, but He simply takes delight in each of us because we are His children. God doesn't value the rich more than the poor, or the strong more than the weak. He lifts up the oppressed; He has a heart for the lonely. He tells the disabled that they are as valuable to Him as the Olympic champions of the world are. No disability, obstacle, or disadvantage can change that. Nor can the removal of a disability, obstacle, or disadvantage make a person any more valuable in God's eyes. Human beings see that worth in each other and want to help each other.

Once I truly understood and believed that my value came from being a child of God and not from what I could do, I was paradoxically freed to see what I still could do. I could listen to a friend and care about her. I could read and learn new things. I could be present and mindful with other people, not continually stressed by a "to do" list winding through my mind. I could pray for others. And it made it easier to accept help from people.

Gratitude touched me when I experienced help from others. It took effort for people to accommodate my need to lie down. They might need to carry a mat or cot for me or do the work of cooking and serving a meal while I lay down. However, their love and concern came through loud and clear through their actions. I felt valued and appreciated, and it meant everything to me. Others were willing—at least sometimes—to be inconvenienced in order to include me. It made my insides explode with gratitude and light—like internal fireworks!

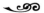

Chapter Four

Reclaiming Ground: Family Life

The Primary Care Giver—
My Husband's Point of View

*A*ndy *is the kind of person who loves to travel. He's been to Europe many times and he knows four languages. He would love to travel to Russia or China, and while we were dating we talked about traveling together. My disability changed all of that. Not only was travel out of the question for us as a couple, but everyday life required much from Andy. Things like laundry, grocery shopping, and cooking fell primarily to him. At times I felt guilty because Andy hadn't known how disabled I'd be when he asked me to marry him. He thought he was marrying a healthy, active young woman with a minor back problem. Other times I felt inadequate because I couldn't help him more. I felt like I wasn't pulling my own weight or doing my share. It made me very sad.*

These are feelings that anyone must face if they are suddenly disabled. He or she will have issues because they need help, and the help they need may really affect the life of their primary caregiver. Both the disabled person and the caregiver need to make a decision about how to view that change in the relationship.

One thing that helped us was to view the disability as happening to both of us. I had the physical pain and limitations; Andy had an increased workload and stress to deal with. Because we were married, the disability had happened to both of us. On the emotional front, Andy was worried and concerned about me but also frustrated by the losses we were both experiencing. On the physical front, in addition to helping me, Andy was working full-time. Because of Andy's increased workload, we simplified our lives. We bought a smaller house than we would have without my disability; we planned simpler meals; we did less shopping; and we had less busyness in general in order to allow Andy to have some "down time." Still, Andy's life was radically altered from what he'd expected it to look like. That all took a big adjustment on his part.

I could still make a thoughtful contribution to conversations, and that made us feel more connected to each other. We brainstormed together on a lot of the adaptations we made. We'd spend an hour talking about all the possible configurations of a computer or a minivan or other household adaptations. This teamwork made it seem like it was us against the disability ... our relationship working to cope with some of the limitations and some of the suffering.

"She's in a world of hurt and black and gray. I need to break into that world with something affectionate, loving, and warm." —Andy Smith

A Candid Conversation with Andy

It is my nature to start by asking questions: What is causing Roxanne's pain? Is there a treatment that can help? As time goes on, the questions become more refined: Are there actually any medications that can really relieve pain? How effective are different MRI settings at revealing the internal structure of a disc? Eventually the questions have less to do with medical details and more to do with the concrete reality in which we find ourselves: If I'm gone for ten hours each day, how can I help Roxanne get what she needs—friendship, companionship? How can I help her see that she is a wonderful person; that disability may steal opportunities and pleasures, but that her core identity, her noble character, remains? And—can I hire a carpenter to build a customized standing-height desk for her?

Along with the questions, there are mental notes to myself: *She's not angry with me; she's angry at the pain. Affirm the grief she experiences daily, but don't encourage that grief to grow into depression.*

I know that some people view me with pity ("Poor Andy!"), thinking that I suffer for being married to Roxanne; and in some ways I do, but not in the way they suppose. Most of the time, it doesn't bother me that we take fewer and more limited vacations than most families; or that I do most, or all, of the grocery shopping and laundry. Usually, I don't mind that we almost never eat in restaurants, go dancing, or go to movies, concerts, sporting events, and plays. Quite often, I don't mind that we very rarely can accept social invitations to go to parties or to the homes of our friends. Sure, I wouldn't mind doing those things, but I can live without them.

What really does bother me is that I can't end Roxanne's suffering and pain; I then feel useless. What drives me crazy is the conflict I feel between what I must do for my employer, for our house and yard, and what I'd like to do for her. When I have to work late, I know that she's home alone. When I should run errands to different stores around town, I'd rather have a cup of coffee and a conversation with her. This feeling of being torn creates stress and guilt.

And I'm not perfect. Sometimes I get irritable because there's a never-ending "to do list" and nobody to help with it. Even though we've simplified our lives, the physical tasks still come down to me, and that can make me feel pressured and hassled. Sometimes I might appear sullen and withdrawn, and inside I feel flat, without even knowing why. The realization that some things—like going to a concert together, going to dinner-dances with the local German club, or taking long hikes or bike rides together—really are "gone forever" hits me from time to time. This realization nudges me into alternating phases of sadness over the loss, and anger over the situation that we're in.

But what I miss most are some of the ways we could show affection to each other. Most married couples can sit on the couch with their arms around each other, or holding hands. Even if they're simply staring at some mindlessly stupid TV show, that mundane event is transformed into a moment of affection. Of course, Roxanne and I do show affection to each other, but not as much as either of us would like. Roxanne and I know that we love each other, and we draw strength and security from that, but that warm sense of companionship that results from physical intimacy is for us less frequent than it otherwise might be.

In some ways, however, I have it better than many husbands. Long before I met or married Roxanne, I spent time thinking about marriage and what it would mean: a decent husband is there to support, help, and encourage his wife. For me, it is often clear what I can do in concrete ways to provide for my wife. Men who are married to physically able women must have to work so hard merely to figure out what they can do to help! I enjoy knowing that when I cook dinner for us, I am doing something that is a real help to her. It gives me satisfaction to know, as I run errands to a few different stores around town, that what I am doing is an actual contribution to the quality of her day.

My main reaction, however, when I think of Roxanne, is thankfulness. I have been blessed with the opportunity of spending my life with a woman who is intelligent, resourceful, creative, and kind. Her character is noble, and her view of life is centered around those things which are most important—relating to God, and relating to other human beings.

And it's not just me giving things to Roxanne; she is helpful and supportive to me. When I was taking evening classes in graduate school while working full time, I often threatened to quit trying to get a graduate degree, but she talked me back into it, over and over. I am color-blind, so she helps me choose my clothing for important occasions. Her health-consciousness motivates me to try to eat properly and exercise; and in many other ways, she gives to me. She also gives to others: to friends, to family, to the community at large, she is a blessing. That people take time from their busy schedules to phone or visit her tells me that not only are they giving her the gift of fellowship, but they also receive that same gift from her. Many years ago I made the decision to ask Roxanne to marry me. I have never regretted that decision. I am thankful that she said yes!

At our wedding, my grandfather read the famous passage which Paul wrote in the New Testament. It describes love. It is a model which was thoroughly taught to us in our childhood, and which we try to live up to in our marriage. We fail—often— and have to begin again, but it is our goal with each other.

> And now I will show you the most excellent way: love is patient, love is kind. It does not envy, it does not boast, it is not proud. It is not rude, it is not self-seeking, it is not easily angered, it keeps no record of wrongs. Love does not delight in evil, but rejoices with the truth. It always protects, always trusts, always hopes, always perseveres (1 Corinthians 13:1, 4–7).

Taking a Leap of Faith: Deciding to Have a Baby!

By 1995, I was experiencing less pain and more function than at any time since my disability began in 1990. I had as much as four non-consecutive hours out of bed on my best days! Much of this was due to the treatments I received from my wonderfully skilled physical therapist and friend, Pam Perkins. Andy and I had many discussions about the improvement and what it meant for us. This might just be a window of opportunity to have a baby.

We consulted with a specialist in musculo-skeletal pain

and pregnancy, along with my regular neurologist. Their educated guess was that a pregnancy would be difficult but unlikely to leave me with additional damage to my spine and discs ... provided that I could have a planned caesarian section and not undergo labor and delivery. We made an appointment with Dr. Charles Leland, my gynecologist/obstetrician. He agreed to deliver a baby at any point beyond thirty-two weeks of gestation, depending on my pain level from the pregnancy. We also met with the anesthesiologist, Dr. Rod Beer, who had done the majority of my nerve blocks in the pain clinic. He agreed to do the anesthesia for the c-section. All that was left was to see whether I could become pregnant.

Sexual intercourse had been extremely difficult for us in our marriage. We had never known a time when pain did not have to be considered when weighing choices about physical intimacy. We were sexually active, but our love making rarely included intercourse. At age thirty-two however, I knew my menstrual cycle well and could determine when I was ovulating by charting my temperature. I believe God gave His blessing to our willingness to take this risk, because after only one cycle of ovulation, I was pregnant!

For the first trimester I discontinued all medication — a difficult choice, but motivated by a strong desire to allow the baby to develop normally. At twelve weeks of pregnancy, I was emotionally distraught from dealing with pain without medication. Dr. Leland rewarded us with an ultrasound, and we were able to see our baby on screen for the first time. That was awesome—we could see the heart beating, count the fingers, and see an incredible amount of movement already. My doubts and fears about being able to carry this baby to term remained, but along with the anxiety I felt the joy and excitement of seeing our baby grow.

Relief was on the way, because now that I was beginning the second trimester, I was allowed to take pain medication again: 800 mg Ibuprofen and Vicodin as needed. Still, the growing baby put added strain on my spine. By the fifth month of pregnancy, I was on full bed rest, using crutches to get to the bathroom. Dr. Leland was extremely supportive of my resolve to become a mother despite my back pain; he sent a nurse-midwife to our home to do the prenatal checkups, and he even made a house call here himself! He checked the Physician's Desk Reference for pregnancy and told me at week twenty-eight to stop using Ibuprofen, because it could interfere with formation of the baby's heart valves, but at 30 weeks it was okay to resume. He also investigated the effects of chronic pain medications on a developing baby. He advised me to discontinue one anti-depressant medication in favor of another one that didn't have potential teratogenic (harmful to fetal development) effects.

Friends and family threw two baby showers for me in the seventh month. They were a much-needed distraction and celebration, because my back and leg pain was very severe by then. My right leg felt like electric current was running through it, and the baby was kicking and moving with some force. At week thirty-four, I had endured all that I could. I went to the hospital to have an amniocentesis which determined that the baby's lungs were still immature. Elaine Cole, the nurse-midwife, came to my home to give me steroid injections to help mature the baby's lungs. Several days later, we returned to the hospital. On April 15, 1996, our son was delivered by planned c-section. He weighed six pounds, eleven ounces, a good size for being born five weeks prematurely. His APGAR score was nine out of ten, also an excellent sign. Andy and I named him Jakob Gotthilf, "Gotthilf" (German) being Andy's great-grandfather's name meaning "God helps."

Since the oxygen saturation values in his blood were too low, Jakob needed to be taken to the special care nursery where he was put under an oxygen globe. I was taken to a hospital room. The pregnancy was behind me, but I was in rough shape. The c-section had cut through layers of abdominal muscles, which support the spine, and my back pain was intense, even with post-op medications. I was unable to sit at all, and walking was difficult even with crutches. Since Jakob couldn't come to me, and I couldn't go to him, we didn't see each other for three days. That was terrible for me, not to be able to be with the baby I had already carried for eight months.

Finally, the hospital found a reclining chair on wheels which I could use to be transported to the special care nursery. The doctor and nurse in charge did not want to allow Jakob to be taken out of the oxygen globe for me to hold him, but we insisted. They agreed, as long as Andy would hold a tube of supplemental oxygen near Jakob's face. The nurse lifted Jakob and placed him on my chest. I just cuddled him and cried, "Jakob, I'm your Momma. Mommy's here, it's okay now." He had his little ear over my heart—I'm convinced this is the moment he knew he was "home." Jakob's oxygen saturation values increased to normal levels in the next hour. That was our little miracle from God's hand. We were grateful that Jakob was allowed to be brought to my hospital room, where we cuddled him and held him nonstop. We took him home the next day.

As we drove away from the hospital, Andy and I felt like

we were stealing a baby. It seemed so remarkable that there was this tiny person in the back seat of our car! We had barely dared to believe this might be possible given my disability. But perhaps, in a deeper sense, we really *had* stolen a baby: we had stolen this precious opportunity away from the pain that tried to prevent it. Finally some of my pain had been visibly productive and I had something (someone) to show for it.

Imagine! We were parents! The first night at home, Andy and I made independent decisions to sleep with our glasses on! We had met with a lactation consultant while still at the hospital to learn how to breastfeed Jakob. Since he was five weeks premature, he had a weak suck/swallow reflex. For my part, I would have to nurse him lying down, since I couldn't sit up in the conventional posture. The first several days and nights, the feedings were a real struggle. I had to squirt some formula in Jakob's mouth and give him my finger to suck on, then squirt some formula on my breast and allow him to latch on and try to suck. After the little he'd eat, I'd have to pump both breasts to empty them. This had to be repeated every two to three hours, around the clock. It was an exhausting process and it took several weeks for breastfeeding to become natural and comfortable for both of us.

Like most new moms, I spent a lot of time cuddling Jakob, singing to him, and feeding him. Unlike other moms, however, I had to do it all lying down. I couldn't lift Jakob, so Andy had to bring him to me for nursing, lift him to burp him after feedings, carry him away for diaper changes, and hold him or walk with him when he was fussy. Andy and Jakob bonded from the start because of this steady father-son involvement. When Andy returned to work, it fell to his mom, Helen, and her mother, Nora, as well as my friends to come over in shifts to do this lifting and carrying. Grandma Nora had just moved to Ann Arbor and was one of God's provisions at a time when we needed help. We saw her availability as being another small miracle from God's hand.

Caring For A Child When You Need Care Yourself

It had taken a huge leap of faith to set aside my own worries and pain to risk having a child. The next phase, caring for our son, wasn't going to be easy when I needed care myself. Andy and I filled out paperwork for an au pair and spoke with several au pair agencies. The closer we got to making that decision, though, the more we realized that it would be too expensive and we didn't have room in our small house to host an au pair 24/7. So we sought out local women who would be willing and able to help in four hour shifts.

We put an ad in our church newsletter saying that we were looking for help. We advertised it as a paid, part-time position. Several friends and acquaintances responded, but they each insisted on volunteering the time and giving that to us as their gift. There were enough volunteers that each person only had to help once every two weeks, for four hours.

I spend mornings with Jakob and with one of these women. She might change a diaper, dress Jakob or give him a bath, carry him when he's fussy, lay him down next to me when he's calm, and help with light housekeeping as needed. To me each woman is an angel, an incredible bright spot in my day who allows me to bond with Jakob and spend time with him.

Jakob is a happy baby and not afraid of strangers. It is pure joy to see him mark his milestones: eating baby cereal and then solid food, rolling over, sitting up. Our home—which was

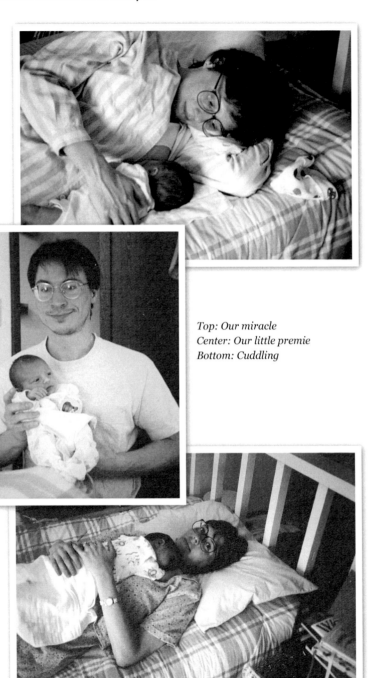

Top: Our miracle
Center: Our little premie
Bottom: Cuddling

too quiet and isolated — is now a center of activity with baby equipment all over the place and people coming and going.

As for me, my heart is changed. After six years of loss and sadness, joy explodes into our world. A child is a gift to be enjoyed and loved. My mind, which has been consumed with fears, worries, and the medical world of treatments and choices, suddenly is filled with cribs, rattles, baby clothes, and books on child development. I am infatuated with Jakob's brown eyes and hair, and I think he's adorable. He looks so cute with his little cotton hats, and when I peer into his little face, he even looks wise. I love talking to Jakob and playing with him, and seeing his smile brings an inner warmth that spreads through me like a warm glow. There's nothing like the smile of a baby when he sees his mother—a huge grin from ear to ear and all you had to do was show up!

I have to rest in the afternoons, so I give my best hours of the day—morning hours—to Jakob. I'm not able to lift him or carry him when he's fussy. I need help from others to do that for Jakob. But what I can give him is my heart: my love, warmth, smiles, and touch. Love is what children need most, and disabled moms can give their children so much love! The other physical tasks are important, but they can be delegated to others. A mother's primary, irreplaceable role is to bond with her child like no one else can.

This is why I think it's important that women with disabilities have the option of becoming mothers. If a support system can be put into place, motherhood can be of huge benefit to both mother and child.

Thanks to the assistance from the helpers, I can make a big contribution to Jakob's life, even from lying down. To start with, I gave him life! My body was able to co-create a perfect little baby whom God designed. Second, I was able to nurse him and give him passive immunity through breast milk, strengthening his immune system. I was not able to sit in a rocking chair, so I nursed him lying down, and the nursing hormones helped us to bond with each other. A mother's touch and cuddling are amazingly important to a baby, and Jakob loves the cuddling we do together. When I'm lying on my back, if someone puts Jakob across my chest he actually positions his little ear over my heart! I'm sure the heartbeat is soothing to him just as it was in the womb. Cuddling Jakob comforts me as much as I comfort him. The soothing warmth of his tiny body against me helps to ease the emotional part of my ever-present pain.

I'm Jakob's primary language teacher as I talk to him about the toys he's batting around or the rattle he's shaking. This "live language" which interacts with the child and responds to the child and his or her environment is much more helpful to language development than "passive language" that comes from the TV. Because of my disability, I have the time to really watch Jakob's development and to know him well. I can give him the huge gift of my attention as he plays and experiences small accomplishments. I can sing songs for him like "The Itsy Bitsy Spider" or "The Wheels On the Bus," and I can do the hand gestures for him.

When Jakob starts crawling, Andy puts a long gate across one side of the family room. That's where Jakob and I spend time together. With the gate in place, Jakob can't get away from me. This is important because I have no way of picking him up and bringing him back from other areas of the house. When Andy's home or someone else is there, we let Jakob explore hallways and rooms, but not when I'm home alone with him. It's in the family room that Jakob learns to pull himself up and cruise furniture, and when he wants to cuddle he sticks his head up over the side of my daybed and we hug. He is a content, happy little guy.

In the afternoons following these eventful mornings, I have to rest. Jakob's Grandpa picks him up and takes Jakob to his Great Grandma Nora's apartment where she cares for him, enjoying a chance once again to hold a baby. Great-Grandma Nora is silver-haired and in her eighties, sweet and doting and kind, and Jakob adores her. He loves lying across her lap on a rocking chair, reaching up and feeling her beautiful wrinkled face, and she indulges him this pleasure. He takes a nap at Great-Grandma's apartment, and Andy picks Jakob up again on his way home from work.

Of course, caring for a child when I needed care myself didn't always go smoothly. When Jakob got sick, for example, I had to prioritize his needs over my back's needs. He'd want to be comforted and held close, and I couldn't do that only in the mornings. I needed to "be there" for him later in the day—or in the middle of the night—when my pain was worse. Sometimes this could cause a pain flare which lasted several days or even weeks. It was a feeling of tug-of-war between my need for rest and Jakob's needs as a child needs his mother. This tension between my needs and his needs carried a cost. When push came to shove, I'd prioritize Jakob's needs and have more pain as a result. But overall, I think we struck a pretty good balance, and I had a feeling of satisfaction that I had something to give my child, even if it came at a cost. The mother's heart within me guided my choices.

Happy to Serve: The Helpers

The "helpers" are so generous and enthusiastic—what a delight to see each one come, ready to serve in whatever way is needed each day. There's Gale, B.J., Helen, Wendi, Debbie, Amy, Karen, Lisa, Meg, and others. Most are friends from our church, where we put an ad in the newsletter saying that we were looking for help. We'd offered to pay the helpers for their time, but like I said, they each insisted on giving that to us as their gift. Each helper volunteers four hours, twice a month, to help me with Jakob's care.

Each helper brings her own unique personality and life experience to our home.

Gale has an adult son with a disability, so she understands how real the needs are and has a heart for serving. She gives Jakob his bath in a baby bathtub placed in the kitchen sink. I can watch from my daybed, and some days I can stand long enough to help wash his little body with the baby washcloth. Gale smiles at Jakob as she puts the hooded towel on his fuzzy head and dries him off. Pretty soon they're both smiling because Gale's joy is so contagious.

B.J. helps me introduce Jakob to a whole variety of baby foods...rice cereal gives way to orange vegetables, pureed fruits, and Cheerios, of course! She straps him into a baby positioner and then a high chair to feed him. If I'm feeling good enough, I stand and help him eat with a tiny spoon. Jakob especially takes to pears, and we can't feed him fast enough! B.J. is a writer and she loves reading to Jakob.

Helen is my mother-in-law and she also loves books. She brings plastic books that Jakob begins looking at and pulling on at around six months. Grandma Helen brings board books, rhyming books, and books with pictures of other toddlers at play. Helen works at the local Borders Book Store in the children's section, so she has excellent resources! We marvel at the illustrations of some of the books, each page being a work of art. Jakob is Grandma Helen's first grandchild, so she is loving every minute that she can spend with him, cuddling, talking, and being playful.

Wendi has cerebral palsy so she also has been sensitized to living life with a disability. In spite of her limitations, she is the mother of four children! She is basically unflappable and takes everything in stride. No diaper emergency or "blowout" can scare her away. When Jakob gets old enough to walk, she takes him to the park which is ten houses from our house. She can sit on the park bench and relax a little while Jakob plays in the sandbox. The only way I can do that is if I bring a beach towel and lie down on the ground near the sandbox. So her help is a real asset.

Debbie is a mom of two boys, and she has a gentle, nurturing personality. Her boys are two and four years older than Jakob, so I look to her stories for a preview of what I may experience down the road with Jakob. She tries to fix healthy, nutritious meals for her family, and she shares some simple, child-friendly recipes with me. Sometimes Debbie takes Jakob to her house for an afternoon if Great Grandma Nora isn't available. I feel like I can trust her completely.

Amy is a free spirit and animal lover. She and her husband live on a small farm where they raise Alpacas, a type of llama known for its soft, warm fur. Amy also loves to scrapbook, which she does as a part-time business. She gets me started on scrapbooking my photos of Jakob. I can't go to scrapbooking workshops where everyone sits around tables for an evening, but I can work on an album for an hour or two at home while lying down. Amy encourages me to write down my thoughts next to the photos. That way I'll have great memories recorded of my early months and years with Jakob. She's also pragmatic. When we end up with a mouse in our basement, she's the one who chases it around with a broom and kills it!

Karen is probably the most enthusiastic helper. Jakob waves at her with both arms when he sees her! We call it his "double wave," which is usually reserved for his grandpa. Karen is a trained dancer and she shows Jakob how to "dance" and "spin" in his jumper, which is suspended from the basement ceiling. He loves flying around in that thing. Sometimes Karen takes Jakob to pet stores where they check out all the animals, a fascinating outing. I am a little envious and wish I could go along to watch Jakob's reactions to the puppies and hamsters. I remind myself that my goal is for Jakob to have my love as well as some of the experiences that I can't give him myself. I want him to be well-rounded and well-adjusted, and sometimes part of that process has to happen without me.

You might be thinking this is a lot of fuss and bother for one little baby / toddler. And you're probably right! Everyday normal events, though, like toddlers going with their mothers to the grocery store, aren't possible for us. Pretty much Jakob's whole experience of life outside our house has to be arranged with other people. Since my support system is a team of people rather than one individual, it does take quite a bit of effort and coordination. But to me, it's worth it. As an added, unintentional blessing, Jakob is benefiting from knowing such a variety of adults. And each helper tells me she feels blessed to be involved!

Lisa is a friend of Grandma Helen's. She is married but doesn't have kids yet, and she's also willing to volunteer about once every other week. She's witty and interesting, and I enjoy her company. When spring comes, Lisa takes Jakob outside. He can walk now, but he wants to plop down on the ground and feel the grass with his fingers. He pulls fistfuls from the ground. Lisa lifts Jakob up to the crab apple tree, which is in bloom. I shake a low branch lightly, and the white blossoms flutter down like snow. Jakob shrieks with pleasure. We do this again and again for him, covering him with flower "snow." Not too long afterward, I learn that Lisa has had a child of her own!

Meg has three children, and she's a pro at getting kids to smile for pictures. She packs Jakob up in his car seat and drives us to the nearby mall. For once I feel good enough to go along. Meg gets Jakob into his stroller and pushes him into the JCPenney photo studio. I feel a little helpless / useless as Meg even has to pose Jakob in his chair on the little stage; I feel somehow like that should be my job. Meg is very gracious and couldn't be nicer about it, though. Jake decides he's afraid of the photographer, and for a minute it looks like the whole thing's going to be a wash. But Meg starts making fish lips at Jakob with her cheeks sucked in, moving her lips apart and back together again. Jakob thinks it's hilarious. As he starts flashing smiles, I find myself laughing, too. Who cares whether or not it's me doing the lifting or posing for Jakob? It just doesn't pay to take life too seriously! We get six terrific shots of Jakob, and what more could we really hope for?

Finally, Jakob's grandpa helps out from time to time. He's a retired engineer, and they love playing with cars and trucks together. They make a ramp by leaning a long board over a

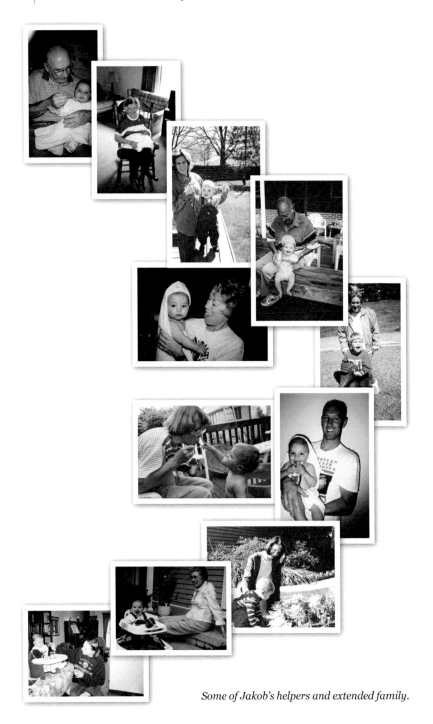

Some of Jakob's helpers and extended family.

low step, and Jakob launches car after car down the ramp to see how fast it will go and how far it can coast. Or they build a tower together out of large Legos or Megablocks. They enjoy an occasional game of hide-and-seek together.

My parents, being far-away grandparents living in another state, have to spoil Jakob all at once when they come to visit us. "Papa and Grandma Lyn" make the most of their few days with us, and Jakob's growth seems very dramatic to them, because they don't see him as regularly. Jakob warms up to them quickly, perhaps because he is used to such a variety of helpers!

Emotional Roller Coaster

Just one thing marred our happiness in the first year of Jakob's life. When he was four months old, another disc in my back tore, and deep midline disc pain was back. All I was doing was lying on my side, nursing Jakob, when it happened. I felt the deep, burning, tearing sensation. The stresses from pregnancy, and recovering from the c-section, along with four months of sleep deprivation from nursing, had taken a toll on my remaining discs.

I was devastated. On the one hand, God had given us the incredible gift of a child. On the other hand, He hadn't prevented my back problems from worsening. Why couldn't my life have joy without pain? Why did there have to always be a price to pay? From pain to joy; from joy to pain. I couldn't seem to stay off of this physical and emotional roller coaster with all its ups and downs.

Dear God,

I don't understand You!
Your plan makes no sense to me!
Look at my journey over these past years
Look and see how hard I've tried
To be free of pain and able-bodied again.

What is this journey all about, Lord?
How can this winding, tangled trail
Be part of your plan for my life?
I want to be free, I want to be well,
This is so traumatic for me!

I know the Bible says that
You will work in *all* things
For the good of those who love You[1]
So do You work in the midst of suffering?
That's just hard for me to picture.
I want to trust You
But it's so hard to see what You're accomplishing here
It just looks like loss to me.

If only I could see this all through your eyes
Perhaps I'd understand
Maybe You are accomplishing things
Through my brokenness

---

[1] Romans 8:28 "we know that in all things God works for the good of those who love Him, who have been called according to His purpose."

That couldn't happen if I were whole
But if that's it, Lord, You need to help me.

Please help me to surrender my will
And trust that You are at work in my brokenness[2]
And that You will give me
What I need to survive

I offer my brokenness[3] to You, Lord,
I don't know what else to do with it at this point…
It is a costly offering, surrendering my will
Please catch me in Your arms
As I embrace this suffering

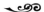

My Three Gifts

Some gifts are so big and so generous they can never be
repaid—only received with gratitude. The gift can be material
or financial; it can be the gift of love; it can be a particular skill;
or it might be quality time. Often, it's a combination of these.
When a person is suffering, one of the biggest gifts you can
give is listening to and caring about him or her. Uppermost
in the suffering person is the longing for reassurance that the
suffering has meaning and purpose; that the suffering will

---

[2] Psalm 34:18 "the Lord is close to the broken-hearted, and saves those who are crushed in spirit."

[3] Psalm 51:17 "the sacrifices of God are a broken spirit; a broken and contrite heart, o God, you will not despise."

not take away *everything* that's good; that the person who is suffering is still valued and essentially herself. Three people primarily helped me to find these truths: my pastor, David Koch, my physical therapist, Pam Perkins, and my Stephen Minister, Kathy Supiano.

Pastor Koch, Pam, and Kathie are all encouragers. When you're going through hard times, you need someone who understands how difficult your struggle is ... someone who sees you in a positive light ... someone who makes time for you regularly. When your life changes radically, and must be lived quite differently from the norm, you need someone who can help you *redefine* successful living.* You need cheerleaders who help you celebrate what may look like small victories to others, but are really big victories to you.

Pastor Koch helped me face my spiritual questions: Why doesn't God heal me? What's the point of praying if my suffering continues? Is God listening to me, and all the others who are praying for me? What's He doing with all those prayers? Does He still love me? What does He want me to do as a person with a disability? We discussed trusting God when things don't make sense.[4] We talked about God's sovereignty, that He is accomplishing things in the world of which we're only partially aware. That although He doesn't *cause* suffering, God *controls* it and can *use* it for good in our lives and to bless others as we grow in empathy.

Pastor Koch had suffered physical pain and illnesses in

---

* My definition of successful living initially was: marriage, four children, working as a physical therapist, having a big house, joining a church, and spending active weekends with my family. My new definition of successful living is: Living the best I can, one day at a time, with the gifts and burdens God has allowed into my life. I will seek God's fruit of the Spirit; set modest goals; reach out to others; and take modest risks.

[4] Dobson, James: "When God Doesn't Make Sense," 1997

his own life, and he could empathize with pain. He didn't minimize it. But somehow he imparted a sense of hope that the suffering would not do me in, that I was more than the suffering, and that one day I would understand completely what I've only glimpsed now. Pastor Koch pointed out that God had given me what I needed to handle living with pain: a supportive husband, my faith, a caring church, our circle of friends and family. I don't necessarily know the answers to all those tough spiritual questions, but Pastor Koch pointed me toward Jesus, the Son of God, who knew suffering first-hand. Since Jesus had experienced terrible mental, physical, and emotional suffering, He knew pain. He could help me find strength and courage to face the pain in my life.

Pam has been a tireless advocate for me, her skills in physical therapy as masterful as her wisdom about how I should pace myself to minimize pain flares. She has worked with me to reduce muscle spasm and muscle guarding, treating restrictions in the soft tissue with manual therapy techniques. She also has had amazing insight about how much to try to strengthen my muscles after surgeries and when to hold off on adding more exercise to avoid relapse. Together, we developed the point system for my daily activities: each activity I did was worth a certain number of points, and I had a maximum for the day. (See Appendix C for more details on the point system.) This helped prevent me from trying to do too much, which would cause a pain flare.

Pam helped me to redefine success—even if I had to rest most of the day, but could attend Jakob's preschool party for forty minutes, that was success! She has always recognized the hard work and consistent effort I put into swimming and walking. Pam has a healing touch, without which I would have been even more disabled. It can't erase degenerative disc disease, but it has helped me cope with the secondary problems. Her consistent affirmation has helped to stabilize my experience of my disability, whether I am functioning relatively well (for me), or whether I am in the middle of a pain flare. She doesn't blame me or make me feel as though I somehow cause the ups and downs. She tells me that I'm doing as well as anyone *could* do with this condition.

Kathie was a social worker and my second Stephen Minister, a peer ministry offered through our church. So she was doubly qualified to affirm me and help build me up. She helped me confront some of the destructive thoughts which tended to recur. If I felt discouraged or like a failure when a treatment didn't help, she said I could not take responsibility for the *outcome* of a particular approach, only the *effort* I invested. If I were tempted to give up, or to believe my largely home-bound life had no purpose, she would talk with me about what the weak have to teach the strong. Rather than seeing only what I could learn from doctors, she pointed out that doctors might just learn something from me. She didn't focus too much on my limits as a mother, but tended to mention things I was able to give Jakob, like time, attention, and emotional availability.

Kathie became a friend to our whole family, and she took the time to speak with my parents about the way they had raised me to be a resilient person. That was very reassuring to them after watching my pain from afar, several states away, wanting to be closer or help more. Kathie accompanied me to a very painful diagnostic test which I was truly dreading, and I knew that she always kept me in her prayers. She also praised me for having the courage to take risks and step out of my comfort zone.

Pastor Koch, Pam, and Kathie actually helped me to receive comfort from God; I believe He sent them as gifts to me, so that I could experience *His* comfort and care. He is called the God of all comfort in the Bible.

> Praise be to the God and Father of our Lord, Jesus Christ, the Father of compassion and the God of all comfort, Who comforts us in all our troubles, so that we can comfort those in any trouble with the comfort we ourselves have received from God (2 Corinthians 1:3–4).

Since I have experienced God's comfort, I find it's true that I can comfort other people more effectively. I have grown in my listening skills and in my ability to empathize with and pray for other people who suffer and are seeking comfort.

Saying Goodbye to Helen:
Death And Loss Do Not Have the Last Word

Sadly, in 1998, my dear mother-in-law Helen was diagnosed with stage three ovarian cancer, and she lived only two more years. She was a very vibrant and out-going woman who seemed to function like a magnet, pulling her family all together, and like the family glue, keeping us connected. When she was referred to hospice after two years of treatments, it was devastating to all of us. Helen was dying: it was undeniable. We were being robbed of this woman, whom we all needed and loved. It wasn't right—it wasn't fair.

Helen had affirmed me and accepted me for ten years,

limitations and all. I wanted to do anything I could to be there for her during her illness and dying process. But what could I do? I couldn't help with her physical care. My sister-in-law Jenny and Helen's sister Janet did a wonderful job with that. My father-in-law Paul kept her company, even sleeping on the floor in her room toward the end. I had something different to offer her: it was personal experience with suffering and loss, tempered with faith in a loving God. We could share the hope of His presence and help in the midst of her suffering. When Helen was hospitalized, Andy took me up to visit her. It was a holiday and the other bed in the room was unoccupied, so I lay down on top of it to spend time with her. Sharing our love for each other, living for the moment, was enough.

During the last six weeks of her life, Helen lay in a hospital bed at home. Andy drove me there every week for an hour's visit, during which I lay on the floor of her bedroom. I told her stories about Jakob, and we talked about our memories. She enjoyed it when Andy and I sang hymns for her. When we read to her from the Bible, she would close her eyes to concentrate. One verse was especially meaningful to her, from II Corinthians:

> Therefore we do not lose heart. Though outwardly we are wasting away, yet inwardly we are being renewed day by day. For our light and momentary troubles are achieving for us an eternal glory that far outweighs them all. So we fix our eyes not on what is seen, but on what is unseen. For what is seen is temporary, but what is unseen is eternal (2 Corinthians 4:16–18).

Helen's faith in Jesus sustained her, and she was able to

face dying with dignity. I was able to attend Helen's funeral by lying down in the back of the church. I wore a silver tulip broach from Holland which had been the last gift she'd given me. When we arrived at the burial site, I looked down and discovered it was gone! That was a terrible moment, which seemed to represent the harsh reality of losing Helen at age fifty-eight. It felt like someone had knocked the wind out of me. I'd lost her and a symbol of her love. After the brief committal, we left the cemetery.

Walking back to the car, I searched the ground, looking for the silver tulip. Suddenly, there it was, lying nestled in the grass, waiting for me. I was elated to find it again! The silver tulip was a symbolic reminder of loss and recovery, a theme I'd been living with for quite a few years. It hinted at the more profound recovery or resurrection in the afterlife which Helen was now experiencing. Death and loss would not have the final word.

> For God so loved the world that He gave His one and only Son, that whoever believes in Him will not perish but have eternal life. For God did not send His Son into the world to condemn the world, but to save the world through Him (John 3:16, 17).

Jakob told us the day Grandma Helen died that she was in Heaven, climbing a tree. Sometimes 4-year-olds have a better understanding of Heaven than forty-year-olds!

> Then I saw a new heaven and a new earth, for the first heaven and the first earth had passed away...Now the dwelling of God is with man, and He will live with

them. They will be His people, and God Himself will be with them and be their God. He will wipe every tear from their eyes. There will be no more death or mourning or crying or pain, for the old order of things has passed away (Revelation 21:1, 3–4).

Helen's suffering was over, and she was dwelling with God. How hopeful. How encouraging for all of us. A day will come for each one of us, too, when we will join God in Heaven. And "He will wipe every tear from [our] eyes."

CHAPTER FIVE

Seeking Medical Solutions While Parenting With a Disability

Seeking Medical Solutions: Motivated by Love

So there I was—I had a wonderful, healthy baby boy, but my back pain had worsened dramatically. When my higher lumbar disc tore and became extremely painful, we found out that spinal fusions can cause problems later in life. Many people have a single fusion with no problems later, but my double fusion made my spine more rigid, causing the discs above it to take on more stress. The disc's job is to absorb shock and allow motion between the vertebral bones of the spine. When the discs can't do that, they pass stress along to their neighbors. I had that underlying risk factor going into the physical stresses of pregnancy and childbirth. Additionally, four months of sleep deprivation from nursing a baby led to disc degeneration higher in the spine. My doctors advised me not to consider another fusion, because it would make other discs more likely to degenerate. So, for two or three years, I was in a holding pattern with my back.

By 1999, a new treatment had been developed by the Saal brothers at Stanford University; it was known as IDET, or Intra-Discal Electro-Thermal Annuloplasty. It was developed for patients whose discs did not rupture, but tore internally and stayed in place, as mine did. IDET was done as outpatient surgery. A hook-shaped wire probe could be inserted into the outer layers of the disc, and heated to approximately 200 degrees for around twenty minutes. In theory, this cauterization had the potential to seal disc tears, and also burn out small nociceptors (nerve endings) which carry pain messages to the brain. With a local surgeon, Dr. Mark Falahee of the Michigan Brain and Spine Institute, I underwent another discogram. Results showed that my pain was coming from tears in the L2-3 disc, rather than the L3-4 disc directly above my fusions. Dr. Falahee said that I was a good candidate for the IDET which he performed on me in July of 2000.

I was frightened to undergo the IDET because it was done without anesthesia. I would be feeling the burning, searing pain cauterizing my disc for twenty minutes. This was necessary so that I could report to the Operating Room team if I was feeling any leg pain, a sign that the probe might be heating nerve roots instead of just disc tissue. To face it I memorized a sentence from the Old Testament:

"Do not be afraid, for I Myself will help you," declares the Lord, "for I am the Lord, your God, Who takes hold of your right hand, and says to you, do not fear; I will help you" (Isaiah 41:13–14).

The outpatient surgery was indeed excruciating, but I was able to endure it. The anesthesiologist was able to give me a medication called Versed which at least sedated me. After this procedure, I had to wear a rigid back brace for about three months while the disc recovered. The IDET gave partial relief for about six months, but no lasting improvement.

At about the same time, another treatment option appeared on the horizon. The artificial disc, which had been used in Europe since the late 1980s, was being researched in clinical trials in the United States, thanks to the efforts of doctors at the Texas Back Institute. For readers who want to get all the details about my quest to get an artificial disc, read on. I wanted to write them down to demonstrate how hard I worked to try to get well. I have to speak out against the incorrect stereotype that those with disabilities or serious pain problems maybe don't *want* to get well. In fact, many go to great lengths to try to return to work or more active lives, or to live as fully as they can even while disabled. If the details of trying to get a new technological option don't interest you, however, skip down to "Parenting with a Disability: The Preschool Years."

As we learned more about the artificial disc, we discovered that there were at least two models: the SB Charite, which had been invented in Berlin, and the Pro Disc, which had originated in France. Both were constructed of similar materials—high molecular weight polyethylene and cobalt chromium—which had been used in artificial knees and hips for years. Both appeared to offer advantages over traditional fusions, because they would allow motion in the spine instead of eliminating motion with a rigid fusion. The artificial disc could bend forward, backward, sideways, and it could also allow rotation.

It could not absorb shock like natural disc tissue, but that would have to be a goal for later generations of the artificial disc. For a patient like me, even this first-generation synthetic disc offered hope because it would avoid the problem of stressing the discs above and below it.

The only obstacles were the restrictions of the clinical trials in the U.S., because the artificial disc had not been approved yet by the Food and Drug Administration (FDA). The research participants were limited to patients who needed a synthetic disc at just one level of the spine, either L4-5 or L5-S1, and who had not had back surgery before. I obviously wouldn't qualify. The FDA wanted straightforward, uncomplicated patients, so that the results of the study could be the most accurate. There was one possible pathway for me to follow, however, which was termed "compassionate use" by the FDA. It was for patients whose lives were severely impacted by a health issue and who needed either a drug or medical device before it received FDA approval — but they didn't qualify for the study. They could apply to receive the device but their outcomes would not be included in the research study.

I also would need to find a doctor who was at one of the sites doing clinical trials and who would be willing to work with me. To find these sites, I needed to do some research. I had been reading newspaper articles on the artificial disc, and also got information from *Orthopedic Technology Review*. The Internet was helpful for reading abstracts of research being done in Europe, as well as early results from the studies in the US. We discovered that the company Link Orthopedics[1] was distributing the SB Charite disc, and I called

---

[1] Link Orthopedics was the American subsidiary of Waldemar Link, GmbH, the original developer, along with the Berlin Charite Disc Clinic, of the SB Charite Disc.

the company's CEO, Mr. Andrew Greenberg, on the phone. He was willing to speak with me, so I asked if he could recommend a surgeon who could work with a complex patient like me. Mr. Greenberg recommended Dr. Raymond Ross of Manchester, England, as being a very experienced surgeon who had worked with synthetic discs for over a decade. England! How could I get to England when I couldn't sit to fly; and would medical insurance pay for a surgery there? We decided to see whether we could find a closer surgeon.

We learned that the Chicago Institute of Neurosurgery and Neuro-Research was one of the clinical trial sites, and we traveled there in June 2002. Dr. Fred Geisler evaluated me, but he was unwilling to approach the FDA to apply for compassionate use of the disc. We consulted with a surgeon doing artificial discs in Ann Arbor. He was also unwilling to work with me, due to my prior back surgeries and fusions. A third surgeon in London, Ontario, told us that placing a disc at L2-3 would be life-threatening, since the surgical approach is anterior (through the abdomen) and the major blood vessels to and from the heart (vena cava, aorta) are in the way. Wow. That was a sobering thought. It could have stopped us in our tracks, but we didn't hear that from any other surgeon with whom we consulted.

Finally, we had my case evaluated at a distance by one of the surgeons in Berlin who helped design the disc, Dr. Buttner-Janz. After sending her my MRI films and patient history, however, she too turned us down. In fact, even though the artificial disc had been used in Europe for over a decade, there were less than five patients who had received one at L2-3, and due to patient privacy laws, we were unable to get information about their outcomes.

Meanwhile, Link Orthopedics had morphed into Link Spine Group. I called their new president, Brian Cameron, on the phone, and he spoke with me once. After he found out I needed an artificial disc at L2-3, he wouldn't speak with me again. We later found that he was in the middle of negotiating a very lucrative deal promoting the SB Charite disc, and that it later sold to Johnson & Johnson for $350 million, which would double upon FDA approval[2].

As president of Link Spine Group, Mr. Cameron's job was to make a profit on the technology, not to try to help a random patient here or there. A patient with an unusual case could only be a risk to this deal, if the surgical outcome wasn't good, potentially reflecting on the product. A call to the distributor of the other model, the ProDisc, was equally unpleasant: the contact person to whom I was transferred was extremely offended that a mere patient had dared to call him; he refused to speak with me, and was outraged that someone in his company had given me access to his phone number.

Doing this research and making all these contacts was hard work and emotionally taxing. When I had to do something especially difficult, I tried to reward myself in some small way. At this point, I'd had pain for eleven or twelve years, but I still was driven by a desire to be well again—to have less pain and more function in order to live a more normal life. Being trained as a physical therapist inclined me to believe that there would be a medical answer to my disabling pain, especially in this modern era of technological progress.

---

[2] Johnson & Johnson would later acquire rights to the disc by buying Link Spine Group, Inc. DePuy Spine, a Johnson & Johnson company, would manufacture the disc. "FDA Approves Johnson & Johnson Implant for Spinal Discs" WSJ Wed., Oct. 27, 2004

Andy and I felt strongly that we should leave no stone unturned in the pursuit to relieve suffering. All the rejections by doctors, corporate representatives, and the FDA were difficult to absorb and it was hard to keep trying, but I had a little boy now who motivated me every day to try my best.

Parenting With a Disability: The Preschool Years

Life with Jakob as a preschooler was fun. Now that he could walk and talk and was potty-trained, we didn't need the helpers so much anymore. Because we had plenty of time at home together, we made up imaginative games. One of his favorite games was playing "store." He'd collect things from all over the house, and I'd make price tags on little squares of cardboard. Socks, a towel, books, a spatula or two, a CD or DVD, a yo-yo, a slinky, a roll of toilet paper, and a harmonica might all be brought into the living room. Jakob would be the shopkeeper, randomly or purposefully placing the prices, and I'd be the customer, looking for a gift for someone. Sometimes a mismatched pair of socks would sell for twenty dollars, and a toaster for a dime, but who cared?

A rectangular laundry basket served as a pirate ship, with Jakob sitting in the middle, black pirate patch over one eye. The "sail" was made from a cardboard wrapping paper tube, duct-taped to the basket, with a triangular construction paper sail taped to the top. He sailed all around the ocean this way, telling me about his adventures. The vacuum cleaner with its hose attachment became a fire truck with its hose, as Jakob donned a plastic fireman's hat. He put out the blaze wherever it occurred, making plenty of "swooshing" sounds to simulate water. Afterwards, he always "drank" a cup of coffee. I learned some children's songs I could sing, and Jakob loved to dance and twirl around to my simple clapping rhythms.

Some ordinary things, however, were scary for me. I was concerned about going out in the front yard or walking down the sidewalk with Jakob. How could I keep him from running away from me? How could I keep him safe and prevent him from running into the street when I couldn't lift him? Andy and I brainstormed about possible solutions. We found a harness at a toy store which had a strap attached to it. An adult could hold the strap and gently guide the child from straying. I put the harness on Jakob and went for a "test walk" with him. When Jakob figured out the harness was meant to restrain him from wandering away, he pitched a royal fit! He let out a yell and his whole face turned red. He squatted down and refused to move for a good twenty minutes, crying loudly the whole time. I seriously wondered whether one of the neighbors would report me as being a negligent or abusive mother after witnessing that episode. It took me twenty minutes to *talk* Jakob into calming down and returning to the house with me. We stayed inside the fenced-in back yard after that unless another adult was with us.

Back inside the house, we read lots of nursery rhymes. A reading expert had told me that they helped to develop patterns of language, and Jakob loved them. When I tried to quit, he'd ask for more. He constantly wanted to build forts by taking couch cushions, bed pillows, chairs, and blankets, and arranging the cushions with the blankets draped overhead. Most other moms and preschoolers whom I knew were going places for play groups and other outings. We were confined to home. What we lacked in physical freedom, though, we made up for in imagination. Jakob seemed to have a naturally sunny disposition, and his enthusiasm and cheerfulness lifted my spirits every day. It never occurred to him to question the fact that his mom had to lie down most of the time, or that she couldn't pick him up. He had my attention, and that's really what he wanted. We enjoyed a very strong emotional bond.

While most moms were dreading the day their toddler learned to crawl out of the crib, I actively taught Jakob how to do it, when he was under two years old. I'd lower the crib rail, and he'd climb over that onto a package of disposable diapers placed on a chair. Then he'd step down on the seat of the chair, and slide to the floor. He'd reverse the order for naps. If there were enough stuffed animals around the edges of his crib, he'd climb in voluntarily.

When Jakob was three, he decided that he wanted to be a pink cupcake for Halloween. It was the first year that he got to choose his costume, so how could we say no? But a pink cupcake! I was pretty sure that this costume would have to be hand-made. Andy got the supplies: a round, plastic laundry basket, to which I hand-sewed a pink bath rug; shoulder straps to carry the basket; white foam for frosting; and yellow paper to make the flame. As Jakob stood through a hole in the bottom of the basket, he became the candle, and the flame was on his head. It was very cute, just impossible to sit down! But it was worth it to see the look of satisfaction on Jakob's face; he'd envisioned something, and we'd been able to make it come true.

The only thing I honestly disliked was playing endless games of Candyland and Shoots and Ladders, fun games for preschoolers but tedious, mindless games for adults. I was so glad when Jakob got a little older and was able to play Battleship, Checkers, and even Monopoly. On more than one

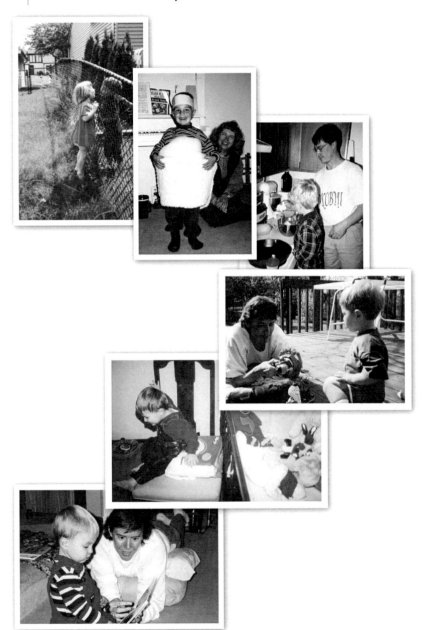

From Top: Jessica and Jakob; Pink Cupcake; Cooking with Dad; Hanging out in the backyard; Jakob climbing out of his crib, as I taught him to; Reading. Jakob was 3 years old before he even noticed that other moms don't lie down all of the time!

occasion, I was Jakob's construction partner in a Lego building project. We built castles with knights on horses, a fort from the Old West, and spaceships of many kinds. Jakob went through stages in which he obsessively pursued one thing, and then suddenly dropped it and went on to something else.

Probably the hardest part of being a horizontal mom was finding positive ways to channel Jakob's three- or four-year-old energy. Our fenced-in back yard helped on sunny days in the warmer months. I would lie on a flat lounge chair on the deck and watch Jakob play in the sand box or kick a ball around. I would blow bubbles for him to chase and pop. Jakob also enjoyed playing with our neighbor's daughter, Jessica, who was very athletic and fun. They had a great time playing in the kiddie pool or sprinkler together. One day, Jessica's mom actually snapped a photo of Jakob and Jessica kissing through the backyard fence! They were four and three at the time, respectively. Our other neighbor had a son, Jason, who was three years older than Jakob. He would come over to play sometimes, too. Jason was always a source of information for skills Jakob hadn't learned yet. He was very patient with younger kids, and Jakob looked up to him. It was Jason who taught Jakob how to dribble a basketball and how to kick a soccer ball. He often had Jakob giggling about something or other that he said or did.

During the winter, however, it was harder to find outlets for Jakob's energy. For a while, we actually put a plastic play structure in our living room! He would climb all over it and go down the slide. Unlike some other moms, I actively encouraged Jakob to jump on the couch to burn off steam. When all else failed, I blew up balloons and told him to bat them around, and keep them from touching the ground. We called this game "balloon volleyball." It seemed that if it had a name, it was more fun.

A great resource for me during these years was a MOPS (Mothers Of Pre-Schoolers) group which met at my church. Every two weeks, forty to fifty of us young moms would spend a morning together, hearing a talk concerning some aspect of motherhood. We'd have a great breakfast and time to socialize and do a simple craft. We got parenting tips from each other as well as the speakers. Our children had their own program for the morning, so it was good for them, too. I had to lie down on the floor during these MOPS meetings, but the other moms at my "table" sat on the floor next to me during the discussion times. They were very accepting and encouraging. Several women I met at MOPS became friends, and they would visit me from time to time. That gave us a chance to talk while our kids had a play date.

We enrolled Jakob in a three-morning-a-week preschool when he was three and four, which boosted his ability to play with peers. Still, his favorite place to be was at home, and when Grandpa came to pick him up for preschool, Jakob often hid under a bed or in a closet. Grandpa played along with this hide-and-seek game, going through each room until he found him.

Jakob Grows and the Pain is Still There

As Jakob got older, I began missing important events in his life because of my pain: I felt bad that I couldn't go on field trips with his preschool or kindergarten classes. I hated missing his fifth birthday party, and not being able to go to most other events away from home. Pain and disability were robbing me of so much. Jakob and I still did lots of things at home together: reading, playing board games, doing puzzles, and crafts. As he was getting older, though, more of his life was occurring away from home — and I wanted to be a part of it! I volunteered in his classroom occasionally but would always have to bring a mat and pillows to lie down on the floor in the back of the room. I watched Jakob play peewee soccer the same way: lying down on the side of the field, on a foam mat on the grass. But I didn't feel safe with the ball down at my eye level, and I felt very conspicuous.

If there was anything we could still try, medically, to give me a chance at a more normal life, we were going to work as hard as we could to get that. I wanted pain relief and a more normal life for myself, but I also wanted it for Jakob's sake. Our whole family would benefit if I were more able-bodied again. I wanted to be able to unburden Andy as well, and help him more with the things that needed to be done. Jakob and Andy gave me the motivation to keep on trying and enduring whatever was necessary to regain function.

I continued researching the artificial disc. The October 2002 supplement to the *European Spine Journal* covered artificial discs, and I read the abstracts online. There were other abstracts about the artificial disc in *Spine Journal* as well as a web site called, not surprisingly, artificialdisc.com. Thanks to my graduate work in physical therapy, I was aware of, and could understand, these types of resources.

During the winter of 2002/03 I remembered the surgeon in England who had been recommended by Mr. Greenberg. I still had the surgeon's name in my records, Dr. Raymond Ross, so I contacted him by e-mail to inquire whether he was still doing artificial disc replacement surgeries. He replied to say that he was. I asked him in my next e-mail whether he would be willing to evaluate my case. He replied that he would be willing to look at it. In my third e-mail I asked about which diagnostic tests he would want to see. He asked us to send him my most recent MRI films.

I waited a month for him to receive the films, read them, and respond to us. I scanned through my e-mail everyday for his name, hoping to see it: Raymond Ross—a sense of hope already surrounding it. When he did respond, he requested that I have a fresh discogram followed by a CT scan immediately afterward. The CT scan would be able to document the tears in the disc and we would also be able to send him films from the discogram itself.

I made an appointment with my local surgeon, Dr. Falahee, who had done an earlier discogram as well as my IDET procedure. After explaining that I was trying to fulfill the requirements of a surgeon in England, I asked whether he'd be willing to work up my case for the overseas physician. Dr. Falahee was intrigued and said he was willing. He performed my third discogram, a truly torturous diagnostic test which produced deep, searing midline pain that rated an eight out of ten on the pain scale. Once again, though, it was the most specific, accurate test for demonstrating my type of disc degeneration and tears. Dr. Falahee did not normally order a CT scan after his discograms but was willing to do that to satisfy Dr. Ross' conditions. Shortly afterward the films were on their way to England for Dr. Ross' review.

We were very glad that the discogram was behind me. Unfortunately, though, I experienced a nasty complication; soon after the discogram I developed a spinal headache. Apparently one of the three needles which were inserted deep into three of my discs had punctured the dura mater surrounding the spinal cord, and that puncture was allowing cerebrospinal fluid to drip out, causing a pounding headache. After lying down for two days and drinking lots of water it had not improved, so I had to go to the pain clinic. They gave me a "blood patch" in which they drew blood from my arm and injected it around the puncture site. To my great relief the procedure stopped the throbbing headache.

We also submitted paperwork to our health insurance company, MESSA[3], to try to obtain pre-approval for surgery. To our surprise, MESSA had no problem with paying for a surgery in another country. Their objection was paying for a surgery still considered "experimental" in the US. We appealed their decision and scheduled a phone conference call between us, a Blue Cross hearing officer, Dr. Elkiss, and Kathie Supiano. We felt optimistic that we'd presented compelling reasons for them to pay for an artificial disc. Ironically, they'd pay for a fusion which would very likely lead to the need for further expensive fusion surgeries in the future. However, we received a rejection letter in the mail several days later. MESSA would not pay. What a disappointment. That was a real emotional blow. To be fair, though, up till now they had given us excellent coverage, probably one of the best insurance plans on the market.

Now we had to wait for Dr. Ross' word back to us on whether or not I was a surgical candidate. I felt like I had been waiting for weeks, months, even years to try to qualify for this surgery. Waiting was uncomfortable and frustrating, at best. In a spiritual sense, I believe God was teaching me to *wait*

---

[3] MESSA is an upgraded form of Blue Cross available to teachers in Michigan.

upon Him. I could do the work required to try new medical options, but then I needed to wait and leave the outcome in God's hands. Several years before, Pastor Koch had preached a sermon on "Be strong, take heart, and wait for the Lord" from Psalm 27. I recalled that and searched for a second Bible passage that addressed waiting.

> In repentance and rest is your salvation, In quiet and trust is your strength. The Lord longs to be gracious to you. He rises to show you compassion. For the Lord is a God of justice; Blessed are those who wait upon Him! (Isaiah 30:15&18)

It was clear from Isaiah that my strength for waiting would not be found in my own effort or intelligence, as logical as that seemed, but in quieting my spirit and trusting the Lord. "In quiet and trust is your strength" —very counter intuitive for me. God promised to bless me if I would wait on Him. He also wanted me to repent and to rest. I didn't know how He'd bless me, but He promised that He would.

On Being "Different": Glimpses From My View

I want to describe what it's like to live life lying down, and to give you a glimpse from my viewpoint. I can't let you experience my pain, but I can let you see through my eyes and experience my thoughts and feelings about living horizontally. This may help you understand why I searched so intently for the artificial disc, and why we were willing to do whatever it took to try to get one.

Being a "horizontal woman" gives a different perspective

on the world. I have a great view of everyone else's ankles. At home we have a daybed in every room, but when I leave home I need to bring a horizontal surface along with me. If Andy is going with me, he often brings a cot so I can lie down a few inches off the ground. It requires lifting the cot, a large board, and a foam mattress, however, so if he's not coming along I bring a thin mat and pillows. They are lighter to carry but require me to lie on the floor or on the ground.

I feel awkward, conspicuous, and inappropriate lying on the ground in public. At times being on the ground makes me feel like a worm or an insect, breathing everyone's dust as they walk past. I'm able to examine dirt and lint on the floor in great detail, as if it were a painting on the wall, having a view that's usually reserved for pets or young children. When I'm lying on my stomach it's impossible to make eye contact with anyone; and if they try by kneeling down or sitting on the ground next to me, it's hard on my neck to lift my head and turn it sideways to have any kind of a conversation. If I were able to lie on my back on a lounge chair with elevated head it would be easier, but lying on my back makes my pain worse and even more so if my head is elevated. I must lie flat, on my stomach, with a pillow under my torso for the pain to quiet itself. Or, I am able to lie on my side with a thin cushion under my ribs, a pillow between my knees and another one under my head.

People do not know how to respond to this. Because I have a little time out of bed each day, I vacillate between being vertical and looking fine, and being horizontal and looking very un-fine and unnatural. What do people think when they see my lying down? I'm disabled? Mentally impaired or mentally ill? Homeless? Someone in pain? Or a lazy person, overly casual and sloppy, unaware of or indifferent to social norms?

Sometimes I am invisible. I am at a MOPS (Mothers Of PreSchoolers) meeting, usually a great experience for me, lying on the floor, as I usually do. A speaker is giving a presentation to a group of us mothers. Afterward he circulates the room and stands two to three inches in front of my face, where I am lying on the floor, mere inches above the carpet. He is turned away from me so he can speak to a woman sitting at a table. I stare at the back of his lower legs and shoes, an intruder invading my personal space. He never acknowledges my presence, my humanity, in any way. I feel humiliated. But I'm not going to let this humiliating incident keep me from going to MOPS. I want to live my life to its fullest capacity. I want to have all the experiences I'm able to have, especially the ones which connect me to Jakob.

Other times I am an object of misplaced humor. I walk into my son's school to volunteer in the classroom. I'm carrying two pillows and a light-weight mat when I pass two utility men working on wiring in the ceiling. "What are **you** gonna do, take a nap?" one asks, laughing. "Wish **I** had the kind of job where **I** could take naps!" the other one utters. More laughter. These men are not maliciously insensitive, just unaware, but still hurtful. Despite these comments I'm going to keep volunteering. Each time I do this it's a small victory for me, a victory worth celebrating.

One day at the Mayo Clinic, Andy and I are on an elevator with a group of doctors. Andy carries my foam mat rolled up inside a golf bag. The doctors see the bag and instantly warm up to him: here are young, healthy people on their way to the golf course, or so it seems. But once we open the bag and unroll the mat we are treated more warily — we're the same people, but with different props.

I eat nearly all meals lying on the floor at home, leaning forward across the step between our kitchen and family room. It takes courage to invite friends over for a meal, especially if they haven't eaten with us before, and a familiar flush of embarrassment rises up my neck as I quietly explain that I must eat lying down and they should all have a seat at our table. No chandelier to provide bright light above my place setting on the floor, no chance to make eye contact with others across a table; just a simple plastic tray with my plate and silverware and an intimate view of the familiar stains in the carpeting. Sometimes Andy and Jakob also choose to eat on the floor with me and we call it a picnic. They sit cross-legged on the kitchen floor with their trays of food in front of them, adjacent to mine. They're at my level and I can see their faces as we talk; making eye contact is an important part of mealtime with family. We all think these picnics are fun!

Lying on a daybed at home is more comfortable than the cot or the ground away from home. The view from my daybeds, however, is always a sideways view of the furniture and the rest of the room. Windows are ceiling and ceiling is side wall, floor is other side wall and pictures on the wall are floor. I have a sideways view of faces, too, and my brain has to learn to transpose those images so the world can look right-side-up to me again. The sideways view gets tiresome—a tangible reminder that the geometry of my world has been altered. Andy buys a card table and pushes it up next to my daybed so we can play board games. I'm a little bit higher than the surface of the table, but as we play Monopoly or Scrabble or even poker, my sideways view gets tiresome. I'm looking across the surface of the game rather than straight down toward the board. Still, we persevere and try to enjoy these games as much as we can.

I get up the nerve to attend summer concerts at a band shell in a park, where everyone brings lawn chairs and blankets in order to sit and listen to the band play. Even in this casual setting, it takes nerve to go because my cot looks out of place. I get comments like "**You** sure look comfortable"—as if I've taken this casual concept a step too far. It's okay to sit on a blanket but not to lie down, because it stretches social norms a little too far. If brittle enough, they might snap. The beach or poolside is really the only place where it's socially acceptable to lie down in public, where people don't question my "ableness" or motives, where I can truly fit in. But the many medications which go along with chronic pain make me sensitive to sunlight and I easily burn, so with a beach umbrella and sunscreen I can stay a while but not long.

The responses of children are the most accepting of all responses. They ask simple questions. "Why are you lying down?" "My back hurts," I answer. "If I lie down it doesn't hurt as much." "Oh," they reply, and they flop down next to me on their stomachs in the back of Jakob's classroom to practice their oral reading. They don't give my position another thought, and I revel in their acceptance, revel in the chance to hear them practice reading. My world spins more steadily on its axis here, where it's way more important that I take time for them and smile at them than it is that I'm lying down. It's also an interesting view from the floor in back of the first grade class. I see twenty-eight pairs of ankles wiggling and toes tapping, their irrepressible energy coming out any way it can.

One friend of Jakob's, though, finds it troubling. "Why

are you still lying down? When are you going to get up?" he asks whenever he comes to our house. I explain that my back problems are long-term and may, in fact, never go away—or at least, not for a long time. He is unhappy with that reality and it makes him think I am sick.

"You're educating people," friends tell me. "You're teaching people about your type of chronic pain and disability; that's a good thing." True, it is good to educate others, and someone else might feel freer to make adaptations they need because they've seen mine, but I am weary of the role of educator. I just want to blend into a crowd sometimes, to not have to be the one who sticks out like a sore thumb. It takes energy and coping that I don't always have. But most of the time I get to make that choice: I can choose to go out when I have the pain relief, energy, and coping ability needed. I can stay home when I don't.

The biggest challenge and coping tip about living horizontally is finding something to celebrate. We consider every time I am able to be vertical, even for a few minutes, to be a victory. There are victories in small things, like going for a short walk one day or driving myself to a nearby appointment on another day or cooking soup for dinner. Society at large may not see these things as victories at all, but my friends and family do. People who don't know me may see me and have questions about my unusual type of disability, but my focus isn't on gaining their approval. Instead, my focus is on setting modest goals for myself and celebrating modest victories.

Perhaps you, too, also feel marginalized because your life doesn't fit the norm. Or perhaps you are part of the support system for someone else who feels marginalized. Take heart! God will help you adapt and find ways of coping which you never may have imagined were possible for you. He will give you strength, guidance, and wisdom if you ask Him. And you, too, can find victory in small things. You, too, can find ways to live your life as fully as is possible given your set of limitations. And then celebrate!

Try, Try Again: Making Plans!

When Dr. Ross read my discogram films and the CT scan, he decided to accept me as his patient for synthetic disc replacement at L2-3. The year was 2003. I was ecstatic at the news; for three years we had been working toward this goal, and it might be in sight! Our other option would be to stay in the US, and wait for FDA approval of the artificial disc here. It wasn't anticipated to come, however, until early 2005, two whole years away. After approval, it could be used "off label"* for higher levels of the lumbar spine. The more we'd learned about the technical difficulty and danger of the surgery at higher levels, though, the more we wanted to choose the surgeon with the most experience. To the best of our knowledge, that was Dr. Ross.

Since I was unable to sit to fly across the Atlantic Ocean, we researched cruise ships that offered trans-Atlantic crossings. The line with the most direct and regular routes was Cunard with its Queen Elizabeth 2. The ship traveled back and forth between New York City and South Hampton England during the summer months. Our travel agent, Robbie Ruland of AAA, was terrific in phoning Cunard to explain my limitations and

---

* Medical devices and medications receive FDA approval for a specific application. They can be legally used in other ways, for purposes other than the original stated use. This is called "off label" use.

to request express boarding and unboarding. She was also able to arrange our return trip, normally an inexpensive flight by coach from London to New York. She upgraded us to a British Airways flight which had "sleeper service" in first class. The seats literally converted into narrow beds, as desired, after take-off. I would fly first class, and Andy and Jakob would fly coach on the same British Airways flight. If things went well, maybe I'd be able to sit up for part of the flight home!

I worked with Dr. Ross's secretary over the phone to schedule my surgery. Actually, Mr. Ross was his preferred title, since surgeons are referred to as "Mr." in England. Apparently he performed his surgeries in two locations: one was a government hospital, since England has socialized medicine. The other was a private hospital in the BUPA system. This was only available for wealthier clients who paid privately for surgeries, or for the few managerial positions in British companies which provided rare health insurance as a benefit. Since we would be coming from outside the country I did not qualify for the government hospital and would need to pay cash for the surgery at BUPA hospital. Mr. Ross did surgery at BUPA one day a week. The QE2 arrived at South Hampton approximately twice a month, so the scheduling was challenging. We finally agreed on a date of July 17, 2003.

Our ship was to depart from pier 95 in Manhattan on June 23rd, arriving at South Hampton six days later on July 1. By July 7, we were to be in Manchester which would allow ten days to meet Mr. Ross and do the pre-op appointments. Ten days sounded generous, but it would allow extra time in case my pain flared—highly likely with travel.

You may find yourself in a similar situation of traveling out of town, state, or country for medical treatments. Or you may be traveling for pleasure but with a disability or medical condition. Planning ahead is half the battle. Consider all the adaptations you might need, and ask for them in advance. Planning extra days for resting can be very helpful, whether you're traveling for medical care or for pleasure. If you have a disability, chronic illness, or a serious pain problem, you need more rest than the average person does.

Meanwhile, we were wondering how to come up with enough money to pay for this medical trip. Cruising on the QE2 .... Spending several weeks in England ... having surgery in a private hospital there ... flying home first class on British Airways ... this sounded like the lifestyle of the rich and famous! But rich and famous we were **not**. In spite of this, Andy's mantra became "It's only money," and his attitude was that seizing a chance to relieve my pain was more important than finances. So we looked at the equity in our modest ranch home and decided to take out a $50,000 home equity loan. It would take years to pay that back, but if the surgery helped, it would be worth it.

At the same time, we made arrangements for Jakob who had just turned seven. He was too active to entertain in a small cabin on the QE2, although there would be some children of that age on board. Andy wanted to be available to take care of me as needed, though, so we chose to leave Jakob in the care of friends and family. We didn't want to be away from him all summer, however, so we asked my brother-in-law Ernie Caruso if he would be willing to fly with Jakob to Manchester once we arrived there. Ernie agreed, and so did my sister Barb. They would plan to stay for two weeks and take care of Jakob while I was in the hospital for one week and for a few days after discharge. We were so grateful to Barb and Ernie for their support.

To make the three-and-a-half week separation easier for Jakob, we told him that this surgery might help me have less pain which might allow me to be able to do more things with him. He was a little scared to be away from us but he summoned his courage and rose to the occasion. This really was a goal for our whole family. We were very proud of Jakob.

Our passports were ready. We had letters notarized which would allow Jakob to receive medical care in our absence, and another letter notarized permitting Ernie to take Jakob out of the country. We bought new, inexpensive, rolling luggage, which had five pieces that all stacked inside of each other for ease of storage in our small cruise cabin. Having read in the cruise brochure that formal attire would be required after six pm on the QE2, we packed a charcoal pin-stripe suit for Andy. My sister Judy did some shopping for me, finding black rayon flared dress slacks, with a sequined black sweater. Because of pain, it was doubtful that I would be leaving the cabin much at all, but I wanted to be prepared in case I had the chance to go to dinner one evening even for a few minutes.

Friends had asked what they could do to help us, and the biggest need seemed to be fund-raising. Several of them met as a group and approached the pastor of our church, Dan Cloeter, to get permission to raise money. He agreed to let them make a video telling our story that would be played during church services followed by a collection of donations. He also agreed to allow them to have a medical fundraiser on the church grounds, which would include a small carnival in the parking lot, as well as a giant garage sale in the gym, and a bake sale in the lobby.

The fund raising group also had me write a letter appealing

to friends and family around the country, which they mailed to the names on our Christmas card mailing list. Finally, they contacted the *Ann Arbor News* which sent a reporter, Jo Mathis, and a photographer to our house. The story was published in the newspaper several days after we left, and it alerted more people in the community to our situation and to the upcoming fundraiser. This team of friends, especially Lisa Maas, who was the driving energy behind the vision, did an outstanding job! We were very encouraged by their enthusiasm and love.

Finally, all the loose ends were tied up, and we were ready to go.

Prayer of Anticipation

I needed faith and I needed hope to set out for England, when travel was so difficult for me. This journey would require a huge leap of faith. I asked God to give me that faith in His provision and care. My hope was that the surgery would give me pain relief and the ability to be vertical more hours of the day. My hope was also that God would use this trip and our story for His purposes. My hope was ultimately that His will would be done.

I am so excited to be starting this journey, Lord. It's unbelievable that You are finally preparing a way for me to get the artificial disc. But I'm also apprehensive, as You know. How will this trip work out for me? We can't possibly predict how my back will handle everything from the motion of the ship to the surgery itself ... and then there's the whole return trip to think about.

I've lived a carefully arranged life for years now, Lord.

It takes tremendous courage for me to try new things, risky things. It's not that I never take risks—like having a baby!— but the risks have had to be carefully weighed and the risk/ reward ratio judged. So often I've ended up with more disc damage after taking a risk, or landed in a pain flare-up. I've had to live cautiously.

But now there is an opportunity for something good to happen, if I have the courage to try. It's not possible to guarantee a safe journey or a positive outcome ... so I'll need to take a leap of faith, Lord. Will You give me Your blessing? I'm asking You to be with me every step of the way; to give us help when we need it, and to guide our journey. We can't plan for every possibility; too much is out of our control. But we can lean on You. We can jump in and ride the river of faith, the faith that says You are real and alive and involved in our lives. A loving Father. A caring Shepherd. A Higher Power to turn to when our strength is at its limits. It's either jump into the river of faith, or stay on the river bank. I don't want to stay on the bank, Lord. Please help me ride the river[4].

> Be strong and courageous: do not be terrified, do not be discouraged, for the Lord your God will be with you wherever you go (Joshua 1:9).

---

[4] Christenson, Larry, *Ride the River: Experience the Full Power of a Life Journey with God*, Bethany House Publishers, 2000.

Chapter Six

Surgery in a Foreign Country: Support Pours In!

Crossing the Atlantic on the Queen Elizabeth 2: Unexpected Gifts

About twenty friends gathered in our living room the morning we left. We held hands in a circle and prayed for a safe journey, for healing, and for God's help. Once again in our lives, joy and pain coexisted—the joy of friendship and hope; the pain of separation and disability. We hugged Jakob goodbye and left in our minivan. We took the next three days to drive to New York City, Andy driving in front and me lying down on the mattress in back. We stayed at the Holiday Inn in midtown Manhattan to be as close to Pier 95 as possible. It was a short taxi ride over the next day. And there she was: the Queen Elizabeth 2. Elegant ... stately ... filling our view!

The lines for boarding were several blocks long and we were unable to find the contact person whose name we'd been given. When Andy explained our situation, however, another employee of Cunard escorted us to the front of the line. Our pictures were taken for the plastic ID card we'd use on board, and another photographer snapped a boarding photo of us together next to a Cunard lifesaver. Moments later we boarded the ship and were escorted several floors down to the deck where our cabin was located.

The economy class room was approximately eight feet square with a twin bed on either side and a tiny bathroom at one end. I was relieved to be aboard but had one hurdle yet to face: the lifeboat drill. We'd been told that it was mandatory to go to the main deck wearing a life jacket and stand for half an hour to watch someone demonstrate getting into and out of the life boats. Although that would use up my remaining function for the day, I wanted to comply with their wishes. We were spared this exercise, however, because we were lying down in our cabin waiting for the alarm to signal and it never came. We heard an announcement which the other passengers apparently responded to, but they were so quiet we didn't realize it was time to go!

As a result, I was actually able to stand on the main deck for half an hour as the ship pulled out of Pier 95. We traveled south along the west side of Manhattan, a gorgeous sight as the sun was starting to set. The skyscrapers were colored with golden light: the art-deco Chrysler building and the Empire State Building gleaming in the summer evening. A tour guide's voice narrated, giving interesting details about the skyline as we slowly passed by. She told us shipboard trivia like how many eggs, shrimp, and lobster are stocked for the crossing as well as the number of passengers (2,000) and crew (1,000) who were aboard. I couldn't believe I was seeing all of this; it was truly an unexpected gift.

We passed the site of the former world trade center and were told that it had been twice as tall as any of the remaining skyscrapers immediately around it. This was an incredibly sobering thought as we scanned the sky to imagine it. Moments later we passed the Statue of Liberty and a ferry to Ellis Island, sailed under a bridge, and headed east beside Long Island and out to sea. It was time to go lie down because my legs were shaking from fatigue.

Andy and I returned to our cabin. It turned out that we had been assigned to the late dinner seating time, 8:00-10:00 p.m., so I was unable to ever have dinner in the dining room. Fortunately, room service was included in the cruise price so I ordered from their simplified menu and ate my meals lying down in the cabin. There was no porthole in our cabin, but there was a television in the room which showed the captain's view from the bridge on one of its channels. It was interesting to see the ocean stretch out in front of us as far as you could see. Another TV channel showed our ship's position as a dot on a map between Manhattan on the left and Southampton on the right. The map also showed topographical lines of the ocean floor so you could see approximately where the ocean water was the deepest. We unpacked, read a little while, and went to sleep.

The next morning I used one of the two swimming pools on board. It was on a lower deck, surrounded by exercise bikes and treadmills and, to my surprise, the pool was filled with salt water. After thinking about that it made sense, but it was a challenge for me to do my water exercises in salt water which was also sloshing from side to side as the ship moved up and down on the ocean. The walk to and from our cabin was significant as the QE2 is approximately three football fields long. The hallways with their red carpeting looked like they went on forever! It seemed to require more from my leg muscles to walk while at sea.

The most interesting thing about being aboard was the view of the ocean. For the first time in my life I was surrounded by ocean on every side, as far as the eye could see. The brilliant white of the ship contrasted magnificently with the bright blue, cloudless sky and the deeper blue of the ocean. And the air! It had never felt so fresh, cool, and exhilarating. Cunard's trademark smokestack with its red and black trim just set the colors off beautifully. A thin trail of smoke wisped through the air behind us, the only mark of industrialization in this natural environment.

Each morning the clocks were adjusted one hour ahead so that by the sixth day we'd be on England time. Most of us failed to set alarm clocks, however, so by the end of the week we were all getting up at noon! As for entertainment and points of interest, no one would have been bored on this ship. There were several lounges with live entertainment every night, and even if you couldn't participate in that—as I was unable to do—there were live lectures in the auditorium that were also broadcast on the TVs. Authors on board such as Stewart Ross spoke about their books and then met passengers in the book store for book signings. In this way we learned about the Stuart dynasty of ruling monarchs in England. We also heard a fascinating portrayal of the British Navy of the early 20th century. Stewart Ross incorporated a liberal amount of British self-deprecating humor, which everyone enjoyed.

"QE2 Goes to the Movies" was the theme of the cruise, and there was a group of actors, producers, and directors of both movies and Broadway plays on board. They spoke about their industry individually and also answered questions as a panel. We recognized Karen Allen from the movie *Raiders of the Lost Ark* who was on board with her 11-year-old son. Movies were shown every night in the theater as well as on the TVs in the rooms. There were live art auctions each afternoon, a casino, and an area for games like ping-pong, shuffleboard, and tennis. I wasn't able to take advantage of much, but it was exciting just to catch glimpses here and there.

In reality most of my time was spent as usual—lying down—but in a cabin that was in constant motion from the sea. Because we'd had to wait until Dr. Ross' decision to reserve passage on the ship, we only had two week's notice before departure. As a result we got one of the last two cabins available. This was actually an historic year for the QE2—at thirty-four years old, its last year of making trans-Atlantic crossings. The following summer, the new Queen Mary 2 would take over its route, and we might never have gotten a reservation with such short notice! The cabin we chose from these last two available options, put us in the front quarter of the ship where the up and down motion was amplified.

On the fourth day of our crossing the winds were gale force and above, with ominous clouds and gusts whipping the sea. Added to the up and down movement was a rolling from side to side which created circular motions in five to ten second intervals, and Andy and I both became seasick. I was able to get by with seasickness pills that our room steward brought us; Andy had to visit the medical clinic for an injection to get his seasickness under control. That day I had to fight pain even more than usual and was only too glad when the sky and sea calmed again the next day. Even on a clear day, however,

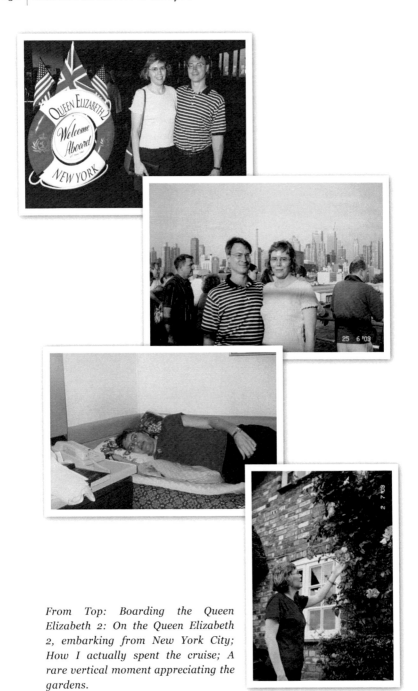

From Top: Boarding the Queen Elizabeth 2: On the Queen Elizabeth 2, embarking from New York City; How I actually spent the cruise; A rare vertical moment appreciating the gardens.

there was a constant vibration on the ship from the engines humming. It was probably not enough to disturb most people, but my sensitive back didn't like it.

Just about the time I would get discouraged by my pain and confinement, though, a few printed e-mails would be slid under our cabin door. We'd given the QE2 e-mail address to friends and family, and quite a few of them wrote to us on our trip. They would be retrieved from the ship's computer, and a staff member would fold them for privacy and slide them under our door. Every time, without fail, they would lift our spirits. The sheer volume of these e-mails was an unexpected gift.

Twice we went to the dining room for the informal lunch where I sat in pain for forty minutes to get the experience of being served from the gourmet menu. That might seem foolish, but opportunities like that are very rare for me. It was so hard to deny myself all the pleasures. I encouraged Andy to go to the formal dinner seating twice so he could toast the captain and meet some fellow passengers, and he did. Many seemed to be professionals in their fifties or sixties who were on vacation. There were quite a few retirees, as well, and a significant number of Amish travelers who wanted to avoid flying.

By July 1, we were ready to debark. Cunard had the foresight to bring customs agents aboard to check passports a day or two before unboarding, and they also lined us up with rental cars while we were still aboard. As a result, getting off the ship was quick and easy; in a matter of a few minutes we were standing next to our rental car, keys in hand, with a porter bringing our luggage and loading it into our trunk. We were standing on English soil: we had arrived!

Letter to Jakob

Andy and I had never been away from Jakob for more than a few days, and we missed him. Every time we saw kids on board the ship, we thought of him. He was so brave at the tender age of seven to let us go on this medical trip. I wrote him a letter during our trans-Atlantic crossing, to share with him when he got older.

To: Jakob
From: Mom on the QE2, while we are apart for three weeks

I want you to know how glad Dad and I are that we decided to have a baby—you. Nothing and no one could have changed our lives more for the better. How could we have guessed the way you would be a combination of the best of both of us; a daily source of joy; an enlargement of our vision of life?

There's no way I could have been a single parent ... but with Dad being healthy and able to compensate for my disability, you seem to be very well adjusted. You've learned to give Dad the bear hugs and me the very gentle squeezes; to wrestle with Dad and do body-slams, but to just cuddle up with me. You've taught me that motherhood is more than a series of physical tasks. One can be a mother without needing to do all the physical tasks. The biggest requirement is heart. You have a permanent, secure, roomy place in my heart, transcending distance or time. Being apart from you for a little while now makes no difference; I am still holding you close.

I may never be able to drive you to school, but I will always make time to hear about your day. I may only rarely be able to cook you a meal, but I will always know your tastes and preferences. I may not be playing basketball with you in the driveway, or playing ping-pong in the basement, but I will be happy to play Scrabble or Monopoly if you want to. I may not be able to go with you to the circus or the zoo, but as you know I will always share a laugh with you. People would probably be surprised if they knew how much laughing we do; it's not just a household of pain. I may not be the "coolest" mom on the block, but I'll try to be one of the "warmest."

You are such a blessing to me, probably because you help me live in the present. How can I dwell on the losses from the past when we're living in the present? There are books to read together, Star Trek episodes to watch, conversations to have. You learn so many new things that need to be processed; you are always curious about everything. How can I be anxious about the future when you've got me living for today? There are school projects to help you plan, Cub Scout badges to sew on your shirt, and Halloween costumes to discuss.

You give me a connection to other moms. Your friends have such great moms, and I get to know these women over the phone as we discuss school issues and sports leagues; which toys are really great (or not) and which G or PG movies are out on DVD. You challenge my creativity, like when you needed a Davy Crockett vest for a book report you were doing. My neighbor Betty helped me make a Davy Crockett vest from her daughter's Pocahontas dress and it actually worked!

You give me another way of evaluating myself and my

contributions. I'm limited, yes—very limited—but you are not. You're healthy and strong, and somehow Dad and I have had a part in making you that way.

Welcome to England!

There were many differences about driving in England that made it harder for me than in the U.S. Everyone thinks about the steering wheel being on the right side of the car over there and the car driving on the left side of the road. For me, the hardship had to do with the scarcity of larger vehicles like minivans or campers, which forced us to rent a sedan. Even with the passenger seat reclined as far as it could go, I was in agony after an hour or so of riding. Added to that was the absence of rest stops along the highways, or any place where it might be possible to stop and lie down on a mat on the grass for a few minutes. I didn't realize how many wide-open spaces the United States had until I left it! So our first day in England was very hard for me as we tried to travel along the carriageways—similar to our interstates—with only an hour or so of function to find lodging. We only had one or one-and-a-half hours per day—total—in the car.

Unfortunately, we never found the hotel in South Hampton where we'd made a reservation, and we ended up driving west on a divided highway that wouldn't allow us to turn around for quite a few kilometers. We came to a small town called Ringwood in the New Forest. There we drove past a bed & breakfast where Andy inquired about a vacancy. The proprietor recommended another B&B that sent us on a wild goose chase through town and back out into the countryside, with extremely narrow roads surrounded by tall hedges. We asked a local woman riding on a horse whether she could direct us to the "Old Cottage" and although we were only a block away, she could not. We pulled into a drive, intending to turn around, and just happened upon it. It was the most beautiful spot, a thatch-roofed stone cottage with lush vines and roses growing into the thatch. Behind the cottage, a gorgeous valley dropped away with a few grazing horses. Even the garage was built with stone and had beautiful ivy growing up the side. A wrought-iron gate announced the name. The sight took my breath away!

Unfortunately, there was no vacancy. So we headed back into Ringwood, getting more desperate because my pain was very bad, and I needed to get out of that car. Andy had traveled in Germany numerous times, and on a hunch he stopped at a pub to ask whether they had any rooms to rent above the pub. To our relief, they did, and we paid forty pounds, sight unseen. It was basic lodging at best: two twin beds with dust ruffles and comforters, but no sheets! I didn't care, I was just so glad to be able to lie down.

Andy went out to purchase a cell phone, or a "mobile" as the British call it. Although friends had advised us to purchase inexpensive phone calling cards at convenience stores, he couldn't find any. He ended up paying more than we expected for the mobile which he "topped up" with pre-paid minutes. He also went to pick up some Chinese food for carryout, or take away, and when he got back to our room, there was no rice to go with the stir-fry. Apparently, rice had to be ordered separately in England. My back was in spasm from the drive, and the bathroom was at the end of a long haul, to be shared with the other guests. So our first day ended rather badly, with me in severe pain, us getting lost, no sheets on our bed, no rice with our Chinese stir-fry, and an over-priced mobile.

Welcome to England!

Fortunately Andy was able to get a reservation at the Old Cottage B&B for the next night, so we went to sleep anticipating a better day tomorrow. We had allowed extra days so I could stay in one town an extra night to give my back time to calm down again. Gradually, we would head north toward Manchester, our destination.

For breakfast the next morning in the pub, I went down just long enough to place an order. The waiter asked what we wanted; there were no printed menus. We asked what they had. He rattled off "Bacon, eggs, mushrooms, tomatoes, beans, toast." I didn't understand what mushrooms, tomatoes, and beans had to do with breakfast so I wondered to myself "omelet?" We ordered bacon, eggs, and toast. Then it became clear when we saw the waiter bring a plate to another customer which had a pile of sautéed whole mushrooms as well as broiled tomato halves and baked beans. This was part of the "full English" breakfast with which we would become quite familiar.

We found a pool at the local leisure center, so I could do my water exercises. After checking into the "Old Cottage" bed and breakfast around noon, we had a "cuppa" tea with fresh milk and biscuits in our room. I asked Andy to bring my mat outside, so I could lie down in the garden and enjoy looking at the lovely flowers. It was special for me and Andy to have a day and night in this beautiful location, and we will never forget it.

The following morning at the bed & breakfast, there were no surprises about the menu, so I mustered the courage to ask the owner whether I might lie down for breakfast. We explained that the reason I was in England was to have back surgery. He was quite sympathetic and permitted me to lie down, bringing me a tray to use on the floor. Evidently he forgot to mention this to his wife, however; because when she brought the hot breakfast out her jaw dropped open. "Well, I've **never** in all my years seen anything like that!" I only felt *slightly* conspicuous at her remark. Admittedly, the British are not as casual as Americans can be, but I was not trying to appear sloppy. There were only two other guests—from Australia—eating then, and they didn't seem to mind.

Over the next week we gradually eked our way north toward Manchester. My time in the rental car was so painful for my back that each minute seemed to last ten times that long. Leaving Ringwood we planned a one hour drive to Bristol, but road construction on a two-lane highway turned that hour into two, so we decided to stop in Bath instead of going on to Bristol. The only hitch was that we didn't have a reservation in Bath, and it was peak tourist season. We'd just spoken with the couple from Australia at breakfast who told us they had been unable to get a room in Bath for the prior two nights. There didn't seem to be any other options, though; we hadn't passed any motels or hotels along the highway anywhere.

Consequently, we followed a long line of cars heading into the renowned limestone city. Bath's downtown buildings were all inter-connected and built from huge blocks of limestone. There weren't many wooden or brick buildings, and most of the stone had a golden or gray hue—a very unique look. I spotted a park on the edge of town and asked Andy to pull over even though a sign warned that it was private parking only. I just couldn't stand to be in the car another minute. I got out and sank to the ground on the edge of the park, stretching out on the grass. A stern sign warned that our car could be towed at a cost of £80 (about $135), but I didn't care. This was one of those moments when all I could do was pray.

"Dear God," I prayed, "Please help us! I can't imagine that we'll find a vacancy in this tourist town but I can't go on. Please help us, Lord."

We had our Frommer's Guide to England and tried phoning several motels with our mobile, but none had vacancies. There had to be a better way. After studying the map of Bath, Andy headed for the Tourist Information Center several blocks away in the center of town. On his way he asked a woman sitting on a park bench whether she knew of a legal place to park. She pointed out a street just around the corner from where we'd been! So Andy used the "park and pay" system which was a black box mid-block that took coins and gave a receipt to place in the windshield. I don't know whether that woman knows how much she helped us, but this was one of many times that we would benefit from the kindness of strangers. Many of the British people were truly generous and helpful to us.

When Andy got to the Tourist Information Center, he inquired about vacancies. The woman asked him what price range he was willing to pay. He probably would have paid any amount, but he didn't want to give her a chance to overcharge him. He said up to £80 per night. After checking her computer, the woman said there were only two vacancies in the whole city, and one of them was available for £85. When Andy asked where it was located, he was amazed to hear her say it was right across the street from where I was lying down in the park! He later confided to me that he had been afraid he would have to make me get back in the car again. To our great relief, God provided a place close by where I could rest. Andy booked the room for two nights.

It was great to be in England but I wished that I could have seen more of the tourist sites. Double-decker buses circulated constantly through Bath, offering narrated tours of the city. The Roman baths were a very popular tourist destination. I was so close to it all yet so far—because of my back, none of that was possible. It was like watching a party through a glass window, but not being able to go inside. Other than a short walk one day, my experience was limited to the inside of our hotel room. It made me very restless, and I longed to be able to explore. But I tried to make the best of the situation. I read the local newspaper to get a taste of local life. Andy brought Cornish pasties to our hotel room which we both liked. It was interesting to use an electrical adapter and to learn that I needed to turn the electrical outlet "on" in order for it to function. We could have tea and "digestive biscuits," which were thick, sweet, round crackers in our room.

Andy found an Internet café and checked our e-mail from friends at home, and we sent e-mail updates about our progress to our friend B.J. Connor in Michigan. B.J. forwarded our news to a whole list of family and friends who wanted to be kept informed about our progress. It felt good to know others cared and were cheering us on and praying for us from a distance. In fact, we had a larger support system than we deserved; more a reflection of the loving, caring people in our church, family, and circle of friends than it was a reflection of us. Still, I think our story captured peoples' attention because of all that I'd been through, and they hoped for our success on this journey.

Once we left the smaller, two-lane highways with oncoming traffic and got onto the north-south divided highways with limited access ("carriageways"), we made much better time on the roads. After stopping two more nights we made it to Manchester.

Although we didn't know much about it, Manchester turned out to be England's third largest city, after London and Birmingham. "Manchester United" was a world famous soccer team, and the University of Manchester was there, too. Apparently the downtown area had been bombed in the late 1990's by a member of the Irish Republican Army. Although there was no loss of life because of police evacuation efforts, the bomb had leveled six or eight city blocks. As a result, there was an architectural mix of old and new as those blocks had been entirely rebuilt. Our hotel was downtown, within walking distance of a huge new aquatic center which had been built the previous year for the Commonwealth Games. My doctor, Mr. Ross, had an office about five miles south of our hotel, near the hospital. His secretary had cautioned us not to stay near the hospital because it wasn't a good area of town.

We made our first appointment to meet Mr. Ross and almost didn't find his office because the street kept forking and changing names, and the street signs were sporadic and hard to see. His office building looked more like an ornate Victorian home with its stained glass entryway than a medical building. Mr. Ross was professional, intelligent, and thoughtful, quickly gaining our respect and our trust. He had me fill out a spinal survey which ranked my quality of life at 54%. He described the surgical approach he'd envisioned in which he would be making a vertical cut through my abdominal muscles, pushing my abdominal contents off to one side, going around and

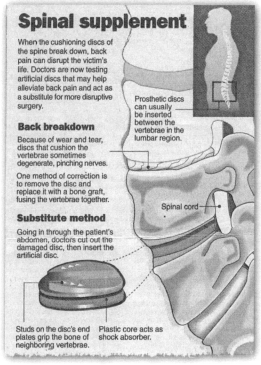

Spinal supplement

When the cushioning discs of the spine break down, back pain can disrupt the victim's life. Doctors are now testing artificial discs that may help alleviate back pain and act as a substitute for more disruptive surgery.

Back breakdown

Because of wear and tear, discs that cushion the vertebrae sometimes degenerate, pinching nerves.

One method of correction is to remove the disc and replace it with a bone graft, fusing the vertebrae together.

Substitute method

Going in through the patient's abdomen, doctors cut out the damaged disc, then insert the artificial disc.

Prosthetic discs can usually be inserted between the vertebrae in the lumbar region.

Spinal cord

Studs on the disc's end plates grip the bone of neighboring vertebrae.

Plastic core acts as shock absorber.

Source: Texas Back Institute

behind them to my aorta. He would have to cut or clamp small arteries coming off the aorta on one side in order to push it to the other side to expose the front of my L2-3 disc.

He showed us a model of the SB Charite synthetic disc, and he let me hold it and move it around in my hands. It could bend forward, backward, sideways, and rotate—or do a combination of these. Mr. Ross was from Scotland and spoke very deliberately and carefully. He was fit and energetic with a full head of dark hair and glasses. I noted that he had long, thin fingers and made a mental note that those are a good quality in a surgeon. It was very moving to meet this surgeon whom I'd traveled so far to see, who was willing to take on a complex patient like me. He was a true hero in my eyes.

Mr. Ross did explain that patients like me who develop degenerative disc disease so early in life probably have cells in the disc tissue which start dying out in their twenties. My disc tissue was very likely biochemically weak. This was another bit of information, or piece of the puzzle, which helped us understand my condition better. My disc tissue would be sent to the medical students at the University of Manchester where they would study it—along with other disc tissue—to see whether they could learn how it differed from healthy tissue.

Having Surgery Two Thousand Miles from Home

Jakob arrived with Barb and Ernie on July fourteenth, and after three-and-a-half weeks apart, it was heart-warming to be re-united with our little boy. Of course, Jakob had jetlag, having just experienced a very exciting flight across the ocean. I remember just watching him sleep, and thinking what a miracle he was. It was terrific to see Barb and Ernie, too: wonderful familiar faces from home. Jakob immediately plunged into life there, enjoying new experiences like eating fish and chips, going to the aquatic center, riding a double-decker bus, and counting buses, taxis, and electric trams as they passed under our hotel window, six stories below. Barb and Ernie bought Jakob a disposable camera, so he snapped shots as he walked around Manchester with them and made his own photo album of England. They also took him by train to Chester, a city with the remains of an ancient Roman wall, as well as a great zoo.

Meanwhile, I checked into BUPA hospital where we had to pay the entire cost for the surgery and hospital stay upon admission. That was a breathtaking experience for Andy! We called one of our credit card companies and requested a higher credit limit—from five thousand dollars to twenty-five thousand dollars—on our VISA. Paying by credit was less complicated and actually cheaper than writing a check. To do that, we would have had to open a bank account and have money wired to England. There was one advantage to BUPA's charges, called "inclusive care." The amount paid at admission covered everything that followed; there would be no additional charges, even for an extended hospital stay.

Once that business was taken care of, I was escorted to my room. Wow! What a room it was! A private room with a separate room attached, containing a second bed for a family member to sleep over! One look at the menu told me that this was not typical hospital food: steaks and fish, gourmet side dishes, wine, beer, and whiskey! I was told that I could order anything at any time by just phoning the food service. Next, the "anesthetist" met with me and discussed options for post-operative pain relief. After educating me, he let me choose which option I preferred! This hospital was quite amazing, and we learned that this BUPA had no emergency room, offering just five basic surgeries: hip replacement, disc replacement, a heart surgery, and two other elective surgeries.

The next morning, I was taken into the "operating theater," and my five-hour surgery began. Afterward I was put into their ICU, where there was a one-to-one nurse-to-patient ratio. I wasn't very aware, but I think I was the only patient in ICU at times. I do know that when they brought me to my regular room the next day, they turned off the lights in the ICU and shut it down! This was far different than anything I'd experienced before in the U.S.

The only thing I wanted to know when I woke up from the general anesthetic was whether I'd gotten the artificial disc. Mr. Ross had said that he would have to do a fusion if he was unable to get the artificial disc in. As it was, he'd estimated two hours in surgery, but it turned out to take five hours since it was technically difficult at L2-3, with the aorta in the way. He persisted, however, and he was able to get the disc inserted. Those words were music to my ears.

Recovery was difficult, and because of the abdominal surgery I had terrible, persistent nausea. I was unable to eat for a week—the wonderful meals which were brought to me were usually eaten by Andy. I was in a great deal of pain from the surgery, and I was very glad to have my sister Barb with me to keep me company in the hospital. She brought me a new flowered nightgown, made of very soft cotton, but the best gift was her presence and conversation. I especially enjoyed hearing updates on what Jakob was doing and experiencing.

Jakob visited the hospital for short periods of time. I actually taped a copy of his passport photo to the nightstand so I could see his little smiling face which always gave me courage. I think that my love for him—and wanting to be the best mom I could be for him—enabled me to do many hard things, and to face difficult situations. On the days when Barb and Ernie took Jakob somewhere, Andy stayed with me. Andy had always been there for me during and after my surgeries, and his presence was always calming and encouraging to me. I couldn't even begin to imagine my life without Andy. Out on his adventures with Barb and Ernie, Jakob got to see part of a cricket match, play in some fountains downtown, and go to a science museum. Ernie was always good for an amusing story about their adventures around Manchester. Ernie could always make us laugh.

After discharge, I went by taxi back to the hotel room in downtown Manchester. Because of surgical trauma to the muscles on the left side connecting my spine and my hip, I was unable to lift my left leg, and walking was very difficult. To get dressed, for example, I had to lift my left leg with my hands. After another ten days, Mr. Ross permitted us to head home again.

We slowly made our way south toward London in another rental car. We briefly visited two castles, Warwick Castle and Windsor Castle, on two separate days. It was amazing to touch a stone castle that was a thousand years old. We had only seen such things in movies! On a third day, Jakob and Andy went to Legoland, a theme park where all the rides are made from oversized Lego pieces. There are also elaborate miniature replicas of famous European tourist sites built from Legos: Buckingham Palace, the London Tower and Bridge, Manchester United Soccer Stadium, and many others. Jakob LOVED it. Even though England was experiencing a record heat wave, he wanted to stay there all day just to soak it all in.

Finally, the day arrived when we flew home on British Airways. The "sleeper service" lived up to its name and allowed me to fly lying down the whole way except for take-off and landing. There was almost no turbulence in the air, and getting through customs only took us five to ten minutes! Our luggage was ready just a few steps beyond that. It was a truly seamless, flawless travel experience, quite unusual in the post September 11th World Trade Center Bombing environment. God seemed to have been at work here, easing my transition home. One thing was certain: many people were praying for us. Andy got our minivan out of long-term parking at JFK airport where it had been parked for six weeks. That cost a pretty fair chunk of change! We headed back to Michigan over the next three days.

Home Again: Support Pours In!

Good news awaited us! The fund-raising committee had experienced a tremendous response to our story and our financial need. Two anonymous $5,000 donations had come into our local church, St. Luke Lutheran in Ann Arbor. A free-will offering taken after a video was shown had raised $6,000. Cards from friends and family around the country had poured in, some with checks for $25, and others with checks for $1,000. The amazing total so far—even before the medical fund-raiser—was around $30,000! This was terrific news, which lightened our debt considerably.

Our costs ended up being less than anticipated. Mr. Ross's fee was only £1,200; the anesthetist charged £700; and BUPA hospital £6,000 or so. Converting to dollars, the medical fees amounted to $20,000*. Our economy-class cruise including return flight for two was $5,000; hotel and living expenses in England for five weeks were $6,000, because we tried to live as inexpensively as we could.

Two women whom we'd never even met had sewn a "prayer quilt" for us. They presented it to me with dozens of short prayers and blessings written on it, signed by numerous

---

* As a comparison, this surgery would cost $50,000 in the US, once the artificial disc received FDA approval.

friends and acquaintances. The quilt itself was beautiful; it had a white background interspersed with blue and yellow triangles of calico fabric. It was amazing to read each signature. We also were told that people had signed up for a certain time of day to pray for us, so that at any given time while we were gone, at least one person was praying for us. We'd seen answers to those prayers, and we thanked God for bringing so many people to support us in all these different ways.

There were also other significant things people had done. My friend Debbie and her two boys had taken care of Jakob the first few days of our trip. My sister Judy and her husband Peter had hosted Jakob in Chicago while we were on the QE2. My parents had driven from Iowa to pick Jakob up in Chicago and bring him back to Ann Arbor for a week. Then our brother-in-law Ernie had flown up to Michigan to get Jakob and bring him to England. Betty, my neighbor, watered and cared for my flowers. My friend Wendi's sons mowed our lawn. Andy's dad brought in our mail and wrote checks to pay the bills on time. With so much attention being lavished on us, we felt like celebrities!

We hadn't expected to be able to see the medical fund-raiser, but due to scheduling conflicts it was held after we returned. It was incredibly humbling and moving to see our wonderful friend Lisa Maas recruit volunteers and then transform our church parking lot into a small carnival. She and her crew had set up a moon-jump tent, dunk tank, live rock band, cotton candy machine, trailer serving carnival food, face-painting, puppets, and clowns making twisty balloons. The Cub Scouts were doing a car wash at the edge of the carnival. Inside the building, volunteers were overseeing an enormous garage sale which filled the gym, and others sold baked goods which had been donated by over one hundred people. It was truly overwhelming and inspiring to see so many friends working hard but in high spirits to raise money to help me. All they wanted to do was try to help relieve my suffering. A feeling of being loved washed over me. It made me cry.

Lisa was in the midst of everything, wearing her cash apron borrowed from Lowe's, directing people and cheering everybody on. She was truly in her element, multi-tasking, her blond hair shining brightly in the sun. In my eyes she could have been wearing a halo! Because I was recovering from surgery, I was only able to stay one hour—but I will never forget the sights and impressions of that day. Lisa called at about seven p.m. after she'd counted the money raised: over $7,000, another $3,500 being matched by Thrivent Financial for Lutherans. Amazingly, our expenses were going to be completely covered!!! In fact, a small excess would be used to start a benevolence fund. We were stunned and ecstatic. This meant that the home equity loan would not be necessary after all.

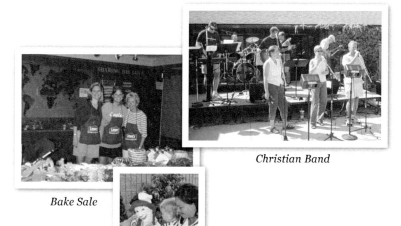

Christian Band

Bake Sale

Twist N' Shout the Clown

Left: Lisa
and Roxanne

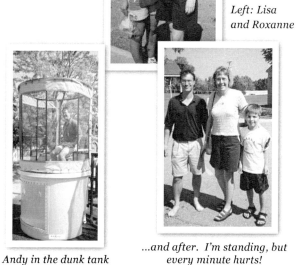

Andy in the dunk tank

...and after. I'm standing, but
every minute hurts!

Celebration and Gratitude Prayer

God, You are so generous
> You've opened the floodgates of Heaven
And rained blessings down on us.
> You led us to Dr. Ross
You took me safely across an ocean
> Provided travel accommodations
> against all odds;
You brought me to the one place in the world
> Where I could receive the artificial disc
From the most experienced surgeon.

Now You're showering us with financial blessings
> Accompanied by an incredible sense
> of being *loved* by your people.
After being disabled by pain for so long
> At times I've been very discouraged.
But then there are times when You
> Pull out all the stops
And turn my ordinary life
> Into something extraordinary.

It happened when we had Jakob
> And now it's happening again
> with the England trip.
It's the year I turned forty
> A year I'll never forget.
Not only did you allow me to have the surgery,
> But you led us far away to England

Satisfying my longing for adventure ...

  For something new and different

To counter-act the confinement

  Of being mostly home-bound for all these years.

Thank you, Father! I am humbled by Your favor.

  Thank you for this amazing year.

CHAPTER SEVEN

Making Peace Through Spiritual Wrestling

The Letdown

After returning home from England, I spent the next six to twelve months recovering. I went through months of physical therapy, doing strengthening exercises and building my endurance again for swimming and walking. Because my artificial disc was surgically implanted at a higher level of the spine than is typical, I had more surgical trauma than the average patient. Initially, I couldn't lift my left leg even to get dressed, due to this surgical trauma.

My physical therapist, Pam, had me strap my left foot to a stationary bike pedal. I could push down with my right foot on the right pedal, which would cause my left foot to be pushed upward. I progressed all the way from having no strength to being able to help lift my left leg and eventually lifting it up against the resistance of the strap. I went from walking very slowly for about a block to being able to walk for fifteen minutes at a normal pace. I started with swimming one lap at a snail's pace and progressed to swimming a third of a mile at my normal pace and doing water exercises.

There was an afterglow from all the excitement and joy of having finally gotten the surgery and having so much help from our church. There was a pervasive atmosphere of hope as we anticipated my improvement. We had every expectation that I would now reap the rewards of pain relief and greater activity. And think of all the things I'd be able to do! Cook for our family, sit up for meals, wear a dress when I wanted to, and be up on my feet without great pain.

To our great disappointment, however, the long sought-after pain relief did not come. Although I was stronger in that I could walk and do water exercises, I still found it necessary to lie down most hours of the day to manage the pain. I couldn't believe it; I was absolutely bewildered. Everything I had researched and read as well as the advice of my physicians had led me to believe in the artificial disc. Thinking back, though, I remembered that Mr. Ross had said many of his patients got better after disc replacement surgery, but some did not. At the time, I'd been so convinced the artificial disc would work for me, that I'd assumed that I'd fall into the successful group.

To the best of my understanding, after speaking with Mr. Ross, the problem had to do with my receiving the first generation of artificial discs. In my surgery, the center of the degenerated disc was replaced. The outer rings, called the *annulus*, however, were only partially removed. The very outermost rings were left in place to act as a ligament stabilizing the artificial disc. On many patients, these are no longer painful. Unfortunately, though, in my case and in a subset of other patients, they continued to be very painful.

I felt devastated, as did many of our supporters. This outcome affected not only us, but also many others. There were spiritual implications to be sorted out. Some people felt that their prayers had failed, or that God had failed. How could such an all-out prayer effort fail to gain God's blessing? Why would God open all the doors for this trip to happen, and not relieve my pain?

I felt that I had disappointed people who had supported us financially in such a public way or with prayer. I felt both guilt and grief at consuming so many resources with such a disappointing outcome. I was devastated to the point that I didn't want to face people who knew me. When I attended church, people would approach me expectantly and ask how my back pain was. I'd tell them that it was still severely limiting, and watch their faces fall, their smiles drop. It was difficult for me to distinguish between people's disappointment **for** me versus their disappointment **in** me. Although financial investment doesn't come with a guarantee, and prayer doesn't either, we all had such high hopes. I had believed with all my heart and mind that this was going to be the answer.

Because of the letdown, I went through several months of grieving that bordered on despair. During this time I needed to write in my journal, to say how hard it was to accept this unwanted outcome. It seemed to me that pain and disability were a valley out of which I could never climb. I felt that my pain would always win, that it would always pull me back down into the valley.* At times, I had feelings of rage and anger at

---

* I would learn how to live successfully—even experiencing occasional victory—in the valley of pain and disability; this is not a statement of permanent despair. This is simply a statement of how I felt about trying so hard to get well without actually getting pain relief.

God. He had provided the surgeon, the financing, the trip to England, and everything needed. Why would He do all of that yet withhold healing? Andy and I had dared to hope that things might improve for me. To dare to hope is to open yourself up to risk. It had taken a huge amount of emotional energy to take this risk, and all we'd done was to open ourselves up to more hurt and disappointment. Was God playing with us?

I was advised by someone who was uncomfortable with my emotions to keep a gratitude journal, but what I really needed was to grieve the loss of my hopes for a normal life, and even to be angry. It's not so easy to let go of dreams. I also saw a psychiatrist and was put on an anti-depressant, which was helpful and probably long overdue. The grieving took six months, and it lessened eventually because I allowed myself to grieve.

At least Andy and I had the satisfaction of knowing that we had tried **everything** there was to try to regain my health. We would never have to ask "what if we had tried the artificial disc?" or "if only we had tried _____" in the future.

The Valley of Pain and Disability—Climbing the Mountain and Being Forced Back Down Again

Existing in the valley of pain and disability
I can't stay here
It's too lonely and shadowy.
I see a mountain up ahead—it looks majestic and inviting
The mountain summit is "wellness;" "ableness;"
Is it within reach?
Read about new treatments,
Apply to several doctors—all say NO!
Wait two years,
Read more about the new treatment,
Try to find a doctor who says YES

I get closer to the mountain:
Clawing, scraping my way
Through tests
Through paperwork
Through phone calls
Through resistant attitudes.
Finally, a doctor says "YES,
I'll be your mountain climbing guide!"

But he's halfway across the world

How do we get there?
I can't sit to fly over an ocean!
Let's take a boat.
Drive to New York,
Board a transatlantic ship,

Sail to England.
Drive to the doctor,
Have the surgery,
Try to recover enough to fly home.
Fly London to New York, sleeper service so I can lie
down.
Drive to Ann Arbor.

How do we pay for it?
The money's all out of pocket—no insurance will pay.
We'll have to take out a large loan.
But in pours the money!
Several fundraisers are held;
Family and friends around the country
Give generously 'til the bills are all paid.
WOW! I'm halfway up the mountain!
I made it to England and back—got the surgery
—the bills are even paid.
Now it's time to finish the climb (rehabilitation)
Reach the summit, and enjoy the mountain,
Living with new abilities...

Wait! — I'm slipping!
I can't hold on!
I'm sliding backwards down the mountain.
Something is pushing me down into the valley!
I don't want to go back there! I thought I'd
stay up on the mountain
Why do I find myself back in pain and disability?
I didn't just want the mountain to symbolize
hope for a summer,

But a completely changed life, with fewer limitations—
A life of freedom and physical activity.

I don't believe this!
After all our effort,
Working for years to find the doctor,
Hurdling the seemingly impossible obstacle
Of travel to a foreign country;
Doing the hard work of having surgery and
going through rehabilitation,
How can the results just slip away?

Everyone else seems to get his or her recovery!
They put in the work and effort
And get what they want!
Other people get the miracles—why not me?
For **me** it's never-ending.
My pain cannot be outrun, outsmarted,
or outmaneuvered.

So I'm back in the valley
After being on the mountain
Thinking the mountaintop experience would last
And finding it to be like mist, impossible to hold.
The best that medicine had to offer
Fell short of what my body demanded.

It's not that the valley of pain
and disability is *unfamiliar*;
It's *all too familiar*.

It's just that being down here again
Is so discouraging, so defeating,
It has such a feeling of permanence
After we had **dared to hope**
That things might be different.
To dare to hope is to open yourself up to risk,
It took emotional energy to take this risk.
We opened ourselves up to more hurt
and disappointment.
We had dared to hope
Our lives might be changed
For the better.

We had courage to try,
And for that I'm grateful,
But I wanted so much more.

Sisyphus? Or the Pearl?

There's a man in Greek mythology, Sisyphus, whose unenviable task is to roll a boulder up a mountain. Struggling and pushing, Sisyphus nears the mountaintop with his rock. Just as he is ready to reach his goal, however, the boulder slips and rolls back down the mountain again. Sisyphus' fate is to be trapped in this unavoidable reality. He must perpetually sweat and labor toward his goal, only to find that the goal is unachievable. Yet it is not within his power to stop pushing the boulder up the hill only to watch it lurch away: a truly futile existence: a hellish, living nightmare.

Over the past fifteen years, I have wondered whether I've become this mythological figure. Pain and disability have had me living in a valley. My efforts to climb out of the valley and to reach the top of my personal mountain have put me partway up that mountain many times. I've metaphorically clawed and scraped, staggered and stumbled with my boulder, heaving it another foot up the mountainside. Every time, though, the boulder has slipped out of my grasp and begun rolling, picking up speed and crashing down to the base of the mountain. What a futile endeavor! I've never tried so hard to reach a goal that proved so elusive. The desire to be well has never left me, but as the years go on, treatment options are exhausted. Surgeries pile up, changing my spine permanently, and the likelihood of my ever getting well diminishes.

So I conclude that rolling the boulder up the mountain can't be the goal of my life. It's a process to which I can devote some energy, but it can't be the main thing. I can still try pushing the boulder up the mountain if new treatment options come along. At the same time, however, I will make a fresh choice about how to view my life. What is the goal of my life? What if my whole life is spent in pain, largely confined to bed, without healing on this side of Heaven?

I choose to define successful living as:

- taking care of myself and the others whom I love
- giving time to prayer
- putting effort into reading and writing
- putting effort into tutoring and other mental challenges
- investing in relationships and friendships

- investing in marriage and motherhood
- perhaps most important of all, drawing nearer to God—not merely for what He could give me (healing)— but for who He is. I'm not going to look for healing as much as look for God's presence in my life, God's help in tolerating the suffering; God's transforming my life, my view of that life and of what gives it meaning.

I will allow myself to grieve the inevitable feelings of loss that wash over me from time to time. I also hope to experience ever deeper joy in simply being in God's presence and seeing— really seeing—His hand in my life.

One of our pastors, Ted Jungkuntz, visits me and shares with me the analogy of the pearl. He reminds me that the reason a precious pearl forms inside an oyster is that a grain of sand irritates the lining of the oyster. It's in this unlikely way—irritation inside a dark shell—that a pearl of great value is formed. Pastor Ted relates this as a metaphor for suffering: that in the improbable, dark place of irritation and pain, God can create something of value in my life. This picture leaves me with hope that God can create something beautiful in the midst of suffering, even as He did with Jesus. God isn't absent when I suffer, He's there. He's at work.

Pastor Ted reads this metaphor of the pearl in the New Testament book of Matthew, where Jesus is describing the kingdom of Heaven:

The kingdom of heaven is like a merchant looking for fine pearls. When he found one of great value, he went away and sold everything he had, and bought it (Matthew 13:45–46).

Jesus is describing life in a vibrant relationship with God. The pearl of great value is knowing God and discovering that He doesn't hold our failings against us. He forgives us since Jesus has paid the price for our sins. This forgiveness is available to all people. There are invisible realities—a spiritual world—and an afterlife which will outlast anything we see on earth. Suffering has loosened my grip on earth and its desires, because I can't participate in much of what happens here. Through suffering, God has focused my thoughts on the spiritual and the eternal. In that way, suffering can play a role in developing my faith into a pearl of great value.

> I will give you the treasures of darkness, riches stored in secret places, so that you may know that I am the Lord (Isaiah 43).

These "treasures of darkness" can be pearls of wisdom and insight which God gives. For any readers who are suffering, remember this! Each one of us is a pearl, and God sees each one of us as being very valuable—so valuable that He goes to great lengths to show His love for each of us.

It is actually possible to learn how to receive the treasures of darkness. Search your own heart and mind to find out what's there: hopes, dreams, sadness, grieving, determination, striving, envy, anger, etc. Feel your feelings, really take time to feel them. Write about them; turn them over in your heart and mind. Then think about where you'd like to be with your inner life: perhaps you'd like to be at a place of acceptance, or letting go, or peace. But you know you can't get there completely on your own power. There's just a limit to how far your own mind and heart can take you.

Then ask God's Holy Spirit to search your heart and mind and to make up the difference! He can take you to a place of patience, peace, or faith, which you can't get to alone. But with His help and strength, gradually you can learn to experience more of the treasures of darkness—the spiritual pearls—which help you to cope with your pain, whatever form it takes.

Spiritual Surrender: God is Sovereign

After much struggle, I realized that I had to let God decide what the outcome of the England trip should be, not me. I didn't understand fully what He accomplished with this trip, but I recognized that I—and others—can't completely understand God and His work in the world. We can partially understand God by studying His written Word, but much of what He does is not apparent to us. God is sometimes hidden, often mysterious, and beyond our perception. It's much easier to perceive our suffering than to perceive God.

In my struggle to accept my ongoing pain, I had to let God be God, and let His will be done. I chose to believe that His purposes for the England trip were achieved, and to trust that He still had a plan for my life ... and that He even had purposes for my pain.

For several years, I had been attending a weekly group called Community Bible Study, a nondenominational Bible study group. There I had met some wonderfully supportive women who were willing to set up my cot each week so I could attend discussion sessions while lying down. We were studying the Old Testament book of Proverbs, or Solomon's wisdom. The theme verse for the year was just what I needed:

> Trust in the Lord with all of your heart, and lean not on your own understanding. In all your ways acknowledge Him, and He will make your paths straight (Proverbs 3:5–6).

I **wanted** to lean on my own understanding, but God was asking me to trust Him—with all of my heart. How could I do that? Trusting God required a different leap of faith than the faith which asks for healing. This kind of faith **transcends** circumstances. Faith enables a person to believe that God is loving and good, even when circumstances are harsh and it's difficult to feel His love. When times are better, it is easier to believe that God is good, but it requires less faith!

Christianity would merely be a facade if Christ didn't accompany us through the very darkest passages of life. God actually wants us to allow Him into our darkest moments, to share our pain and emotional anguish with Him. He accepts every emotion, even our anger. He stands ready to suffer alongside[*] us. Hope is born in our hearts when we realize that we are not alone; that God will never abandon us. Hope is nurtured by the realization that the presence of God will give us strength to face our suffering, one day at a time. This kind of hope is not dependent upon a change in external circumstances.

If suffering is like being caught in a maze, initially the goal is to find your way out of the maze. If years go by and prayers for an escape are answered with a "No", "Wait", "Trust Me" or "My timing is not yet here," you can choose to change your goal. Rather than expending all your energy trying to get out

---

[*] This He did most deeply, completely, and effectively in Jesus.

of the maze, you can choose to accept being in the maze, and allow God to use that maze to make you more Christ-like. God can sculpt your character to His will and desires if you submit to the discipline of the maze, even to its confinement and frustrations. Perhaps there are even some beautiful places in the maze that you'll discover. And one day, you may find yourself at the exit from the maze, given the gift of freedom once again, even though that hasn't been your primary goal.

Eventually, I reached a new level of acceptance. My life was not my own; it belonged to God. If pain and disability were a valley, God would walk through that valley with me. I had memorized Psalm 23— "The Lord is my Shepherd" —as a child, and Andy reminded me of the section "When I walk through the valley of the shadow of death [and pain], I will fear no evil, for You are with me." By inserting the phrase "and pain," Andy pointed me to a very meaningful and personal application of Psalm 23. Yes, pain did drag me back again into that valley. But Jesus met me there. I chose to accept the life God had given me, and to offer it back to Him as a sacrificial act of worship.[1]

I learned that whether God chooses to relieve suffering, or whether suffering continues, He is at work. He is at work when He relieves suffering, and He is at work when suffering continues—He works in, around, and through suffering.

And that's how I found peace and acceptance in the midst of ongoing suffering. Every day I have to strive to find that peace again, because it doesn't just come and stay. The exercise of faith is what brings peace. I have to exercise it. My

---

[1] Veith, Gene. *The Spirituality of the Cross*. St. Louis, Missouri: Concordia Publishing House 1999.

goal is to be a faithful follower of God, whether He heals me or not. God is the potter; I am the clay. Does the pot tell the potter how to craft the clay?

There are two important characteristics about God: He is sovereign, and He loves me. I can't control God or make Him remove my suffering, although He may choose to do so. But I can count on His love for me, and that He won't abandon or forsake me. His thoughts and ways are complex, encompassing all the past, all the future, and the billions of people on the planet.

> "For my thoughts are not your thoughts, neither are your ways my ways," declares the Lord. "As the heavens are higher than the earth, so are my ways higher than your ways, and my thoughts than your thoughts" (Isaiah 55:8–9).

My thoughts and ways encompass a very small part of time and space. We have different points of view, God and I. From my point of view, suffering looks non-productive, but from God's point of view, it may be very productive. Jesus accomplished our salvation through suffering on the cross. Jesus has experienced my brokenness and more. Jesus understands the pain, the isolation, the sorrow, and the loneliness. What's more, Jesus is here suffering it with me. He feels my pain, and gives me the strength I need to bear it.

> For great is your love, higher than the heavens; your faithfulness reaches to the skies (Psalm 108:4).

God pairs His power with love. Love is at the core of God's

sovereignty. If His thoughts are as high as the heavens, so is His love. It may sound presumptuous to say, that the God of the universe wants my company, but what He wants most from me is me ... and that I would crave His presence above all else. And God wants not only my company, but the company of all of His children. He doesn't just want this from us, but He wants this for us. I can trust a God like that. I can surrender my will to His.

And that's a form of spiritual healing.

CHAPTER EIGHT

Jakob Grows Up as God Molds a Child

Jakob's Essay

Jakob has been aware that I am writing this book, and he knows that Andy's perspective is represented. I asked him if he would like to have his viewpoint recorded, too, and he willingly agreed. I want to give Jakob a chance to express the effects in a child's life of having a parent who is disabled. So, these are his words:

Hi. I'm Jakob. I am twelve years old. These are some of the changes in my life because of my mom's disability. Before I was born, my mom got severe back pain. Because of her pain, she must lie down and rarely get up. She takes lots of medication to try to make her pain gentler. Sometimes she goes swimming or mall walking in the mornings, but the rest of the day she has to lie down on a daybed. She can't usually do many things around the house.

I like to do things with my mom. We play board games and sometimes work on homework together, while she's lying down. She likes to listen to me practicing the piano and clarinet. Last summer she taught me how to type when I got my new laptop. She was lying down on her daybed, and I sat right next to her, and she told me where the letters were on the keyboard. My mom can't drive me anywhere, or stand up and walk around for more than half an hour. I wish that Mom could sit and stand. I wish that she could play games that involve standing up and moving around, like ping-pong and tennis. I wish she could go to certain events, too, like when there's a concert I'm in, or a game I'm playing in, I wish she could be there. She wants to come to my activities, but she can't.

I don't like it that my mom has limits, and I wish that she could go places and do things with me. But I'm close to my mom, and she tries to be nice to me 99.9% of the time.

Some good things have come out of my mom's disability. She can be home with me when I'm sick and I can't go to school. She's not too busy to spend time with me. And she lets me have friends over because she's almost always home. I got to go to England when I was seven because she had surgery there. I have learned some things from watching my mom deal with her pain, like courage, and how to face hard things and endure them.

It all affects my dad, too. He has to take me to places I have to go, like to school and Boy Scouts and piano lessons and sports. He has to do errands and other things. Actually, he does a lot around the house, like laundry, mowing the lawn, doing the dishes, and going grocery shopping. I don't think Dad is upset that he has to do so much work. If he were, you wouldn't know it, because he doesn't complain about it. Instead, he does it cheerfully. I've learned things from watching my dad. I've learned how to serve other people and help other people when they can't do things—with joy, and not complaining.

I have a friend who also has a family member with a disability. His name is David, and his sister is in a wheelchair and she can't talk. His brother has cerebral palsy. It helps me to know this family, because I know I'm not the only one with someone I love who can't do most things that other people can.

I know that God loves me and my parents. We prayed for God to heal mom's back, but she's still disabled. I wish God would heal her. But even if He doesn't, I know He cares about our family, even though my mom suffers with pain. He gives me lots of other blessings, and He sent Jesus to die for me and to save me from my sins and death.

I usually have to do chores and other things around the house, like lifting the milk gallons, carrying Mom's stuff and helping Dad in the yard. I have to fold and put away my laundry, and I usually have to put Mom's chaise lounge cushion out on the deck if my dad's not home. Sometimes I don't feel like doing all that, but I know I'm helping Mom and she doesn't have to hurt her back to get it done.

Summary by Kathie Supiano

I feel honored to contribute my observations on Roxanne and Andy's desire to have a child under their circumstances, but I must immediately acknowledge that I was not involved in those early days. In our large congregation, I only knew of their situation from afar, and as a working mom, was not in that circle of saints who nurtured both Roxanne and Jakob in his infancy.

Yet, to imagine what it must have been like for them to decide to have a baby! Having a child is a faith statement for all parents. Even when our hearts burn with confidence that all will go well, most of us as prospective parents have doubts about how we will manage. Knowing the challenges of getting though each day alone, the prospect of bringing a completely dependent infant into the world must have been daunting. For Roxanne and Andy though, the acceptance of the freely given care of so many loving women must have been an amazing experience. Roxi's background and temperament are not unlike my own. So I am certain that receiving so much assistance, knowing she could never repay it in the usual sense of the word, must have been somewhat off putting. God's remarkable invitation to her; "have the grace to receive," has, in my view, greatly shaped her acceptance of her limitations.

It's easy in hindsight to make statements like, "the receiver gives back in appreciation", or "the giver receives in grace and satisfaction".... all true; but like most Christians, and nearly all Christian women, Roxi is more comfortable in the role of "giver" than "receiver." This is true for all of us; we feel more "Christ-like" as giver, but in truth, we also experience a bit of power and superiority in that role, whether we seek it or not. Roxanne was able to capture another side of Jesus in her acceptance of these gifts, to connect with Jesus in His few moments when others ministered to Him. Remember, Jesus too had his small circle of loving women who traveled with

Him and attended to His needs.

And what of Jakob? One of my delights in having Roxanne as a friend is to have been able to watch Jakob in his school years. Would Andy and Roxanne have wanted Jakob to have the life of any other kid? Certainly. But the Lord had a different plan for Jakob as well. Even as a very small guy, Jakob was gentle and patient. In his normal developmental moments of defiance, he would still yield to his mother's needs as soon as they became apparent to him. Those of you who have raised boys can recall the continuous motion, the unrelenting curiosity and the knack of getting into things that boys possess! Imagine the toddler who wants to climb up on his mother or be lifted, the preschooler who runs circles in the house and bounces on the beds, the school age child who must respect limits of house and yard when out of his mother's field of vision. In Jakob's case, his curiosity was directed into amazing lego constructions, and trains that wound through the house. His socialization into having kids over to his house, and adhering to the rules of safety for his mom. And, the sadness of so many school activities, birthday parties, scout events, baseball and basketball games without his mom present to cheer him on.

Jakob has become a young man who is highly internally directed. He can cook a simple meal from instructions given from Roxi in the living room. He uses his computer time well, and he can focus on piano practice and homework. He has developed a "narrative ability" well beyond his years; sharing all of the details of his outings with Roxanne, so she can participate vicariously. Most importantly, Jakob is becoming a remarkably empathetic and compassionate young man. He is highly sensitive to his mother's situation. Of course he balks on the demands for maturity on occasions, but it is extraordinary to see how respectful, loving and deferential Jakob is to his mom's needs. You will be pleased to know, that Jakob is no little angel ... I have seen plenty of sneaky tricks and a good bit of wrestling with neighbor boys in the family room! But overall, his young conscience is dead-on accurate. It has seemed such a wonderful demonstration of how God uses adversity to shape the natural gifts He has endowed us with, and I often wonder how God will use Jakob as an adult.

When I reflect on Roxanne and Andy as parents, I find myself grateful for their example in my life, even though my children are older than Jakob. God takes our responsibility as parents very seriously, and He allows us not only to "co-create" with Him, but to model ourselves after His Fatherhood. Other limitations have been placed on Roxanne's life: she is unable to "work" in the world of employment. This job of parenting, however, though still unfinished in Jakob, has been a calling that Andy and Roxi have responded to with love and submission.

Jakob and Andy: Father-Son Relationship

As Jakob gets older, our family life is changing; it's less home-based than it used to be. Since Jakob was in first grade, Andy and I have encouraged him to be involved in activities outside of school. He began Cub Scouts in second grade, and he added baseball and piano lessons in third. In fourth grade, Jakob played volleyball, basketball, and baseball. He went to Sunday school and to a couple of three-day camps. He continued with piano lessons and Scouts. At the time of this writing, Jakob is in sixth grade. He ran cross-country in the fall, and he chose the clarinet for his band instrument. After a few weeks of school, he told me, "Mom, I was born to play the clarinet!" The same lungs that got a work-out in cross-country also got a work-out in band!

Jakob is really thriving on these activities and building confidence and competence in many new skills. I find myself cheering him on from a distance, only hearing about these activities when Andy and Jakob walk in the door afterwards. Naturally, I encourage Andy to be part of these opportunities, as a Cub Scout dad and volleyball assistant coach, a Sunday school teacher and a parent driver/chaperone for the camps. But it takes something from me to let them go out to these activities. I feel a physical loss.

I find I miss out on seeing them in these varied environments, on being there to see Jakob's excitement as he scores a point in volleyball or his happiness at receiving a badge at his Cub Scout pack meeting. I miss seeing Andy in these different roles with Jakob, and find myself more than a little envious. I long to be one of the parents sitting on bleachers watching the game. I want to see the kids on the team interacting, and chat with the other moms. Instead, I spend another afternoon or evening at home, lying down, in pain. I struggle with confinement and boredom. I wrestle with the knowledge that Jakob is only young once, and I'm missing so much of his life. I'd like to go on a field trip—just once!— and be part of life with its color and emotion, reality and even turbulence. Events which should or could be family outings, become father-son outings.

Andy tries to describe his outings with Jakob to fill in some of the missing pieces for me. I look forward to his narratives, clinging to every detail he gives up, trying to picture in my mind the sound of the fans at the game, the smell of the hotdogs at the cookout.

Jake, Andy tells me, using our familiar nickname for our son, rarely wants to get in the car to go somewhere, but by the time he arrives at the destination he's enthusiastic about what they've come to do. Andy laughs as he tells me about the pranks Jake and the other Cub Scouts play on each other, themselves laughing with boyish glee at their own cleverness. He tells me Jake took out Matthew in a wrestling match tonight on the den leader's living room floor and then later they hid from the other boys in the basement. It's a wonder they get anything done! But Andy tells me that they did manage to work toward one of their badges, and when one of the older scouts demonstrated an advanced skill, Jake really soaked it in.

Andy tells me that at baseball practice, the kids on Jake's team, the Lawton Lynx, alternate between the frustration of striking out and the elation of a good hit. Last year's coach-pitch baseball gave the boys a fairly reliable target to swing at. This year, as the boys begin to pitch for each other, it's impossible to predict where the ball will wind up! Maybe across the plate, maybe way off.

Andy reports that before golf lessons in the junior league, Jakob sits quietly next to him until he sees Josh. Then they become animated and the two of them run off to practice putting. At the end of last summer's league play, Jake and Andy could go play a round of golf—just the two of them—on a par three course. Andy said that Jake did very well and practically burst out of his skin when he made par on a hole. That was a really fun way for the two of them to spend an afternoon.

Finally, Andy tells me about a number of spectator events that they've enjoyed. The University of Michigan is practically in our back yard, so they've seen U of M's basketball, baseball, hockey, and volleyball teams. Hockey crowds are wild, but Jakob and Andy tell me that a volleyball crowd is rowdier than I might expect! Andy says that sometimes it's hard to tell whether Jakob is having more fun cheering for the team or buying another pretzel or bag of popcorn. He seems to enjoy both! Jakob has become a serious Michigan fan—Andy's *alma mater*.

I'm happy for Andy and Jakob, and I honestly wouldn't have it any other way for them. I just wish wish wish wish wish wish WISH **WISH** I could do those things, too! As I continue to write, the world continues to turn on its axis. Seasons come and go, and with spring my restlessness always increases. From my daybed in the living room I watch people through the window. They're riding bikes, gardening, taking walks, pushing strollers. Andy and Jakob are shooting hoops in the driveway, tossing a baseball around, or doing landscaping projects together.

Inside the house, I am watching them. Somewhere within me there's still a twenty-year-old young woman who is dying to join them, to dribble the basketball and shoot, to play croquet in the yard, to hop on a bike and ride twenty miles with them. Somewhere within me, there's an undeniable longing to move with freedom and without pain, to engage in active life. Oh, it's so hard to be patient! It's so hard to want them to have abilities and experiences which are out of reach for me. It strains my self-control, and I feel as though I'm going to jump right out of my skin. If I had to lose the active life, at least I should have been given the ability to stand still or to sit up.

But that has been taken away, too, so I must be a spectator from lying down on my daybed.

By God's grace, however, I haven't lost sight of the importance of supporting a balanced life for Andy and Jakob. I haven't sunk to the depth of insisting that they never do anything I can't do or that they never leave me at home alone. By God's grace, I can want what's best for them, even though it's sometimes lonely for me ... even though it requires self-sacrifice. I know that my sacrifices are contributing to Jakob developing in a healthy and normal way, and not being emotionally crippled because of my disability. That's an important source of motivation for me. I want Jakob to be as healthy in every way as is possible.

Andy and Jakob are heading off to a baseball game, fireworks, and a sleepover on the outfield of a minor league team Friday. I'd love to be able to do that with them. But it isn't possible. They recently went to an adventure camp together which had horseback riding, wall climbing, and lots of indoor games. They also went to a rocket camp together where they built and fired off a rocket. The abundance of opportunities and activities available to them is amazing.

I know, too, that it's important for boys to separate from their mothers in early adolescence. I realize that Jakob needs to learn masculinity from Andy and other men. There are definitely benefits for both of them in spending this time together, and Jakob's development couldn't proceed normally without it. Andy can pass on his values, views, and much life experience in this way. They can make memories for the future. They can just have fun together! I don't want to take anything away from them. I'm only saying that I wish I could come along *some* of the time. I wish I could go to a play or

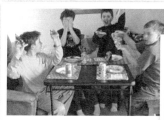

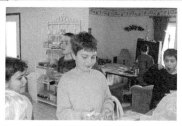

Jakob's birthday party

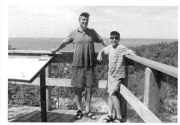

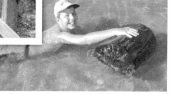

Fun at Lake Michigan

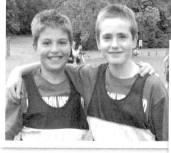

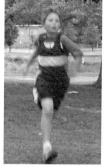

*Above: Good friends and team
mates.
Right: Cross country meet.*

concert or a ball game Jakob's in. I wish I had enough function to go along on a day trip to a museum …

"Yes, this is the airplane that Uncle Steve flew in Vietnam." Andy and Jakob pause in front of the steel-plated aircraft in the museum in Dayton, Ohio. They've driven down to the Wright-Patterson Air Force Museum for the day. The plane is a cargo plane, boxy and silver like an Air-Stream trailer with wings. It looks out of place in a line of sleek-looking jets. The cargo plane was what the Air Force used in Viet Nam to spray Agent Orange, defoliating parts of the jungle.

"Too bad Mom couldn't have come along to see this. She always calls Uncle Steve on Veteran's Day." Andy and Jakob are subdued as they try to imagine the cargo plane being shot down by the Viet Cong. They try to visualize Uncle Steve patching it up enough to get it flying again, before the enemy closed in. They read the sign that says this particular plane is nicknamed "Patches" because it took over one thousand bullets, more than any plane in the war. They shake their heads because words can't express their feelings.

As they amble further through the displays, Andy's cell phone rings. Roxanne is calling simply to say "Hi!" and see how their day is going. They each give her a summary of what they've seen and done so far. Static and a weak signal bring the conversation to a premature end. "We'd better hang up now, I can barely hear you."

Andy and Jakob walk on slowly in silence, both thinking the same thing: It's sad that she can't be with us on this little excursion today. She belongs here with us.

During the car ride home, they play the alphabet game, trying to find the letters of the alphabet in order on roadside billboards as they cruise down the interstate. They play the game, but conclude: "It's not as much fun when Mom's not here."

Later, at home, Andy loads digital pictures onto the laptop. He sets the computer on Roxanne's daybed, where she advances through the pictures of her brother's plane. She tries to visualize bullets ripping through the metal with Steve inside—so traumatic, it makes tears well up in her eyes. And, surprisingly, anger—at the size of the cargo area being so large. "They couldn't have given the Viet Cong a better target if they'd tried," Roxanne states emphatically. "Between flying low and flying slow, it was like giving the enemy target practice."

Anger—and then sadness—that Steve has had to carry psychological wounds and post-traumatic stress disorder ever since. If only he could have been spared such suffering. It's so tragic and unfair. And then—the thought that Roxanne isn't the only one in the family with a disability. Disabilities come in many forms. Somehow it helps to know this. Roxanne would never wish suffering on anyone else, but in light of the fact that suffering does happen, it helps to know there are other people facing it and living courageously with it.

Despite the fact that I can't go on these trips with Andy and Jakob, there still are activities that are home-based: playing cards, reading together, being silly and laughing, just having conversations. In some ways, our family has a rich home life. We're intentional about spending quality time together, and we value close relationships with each other. Because we've simplified our lives in response to my disability, we actually have a couple of hours on Sunday afternoon to play Monopoly or Star Wars LIFE together. We enjoy watching movies at home as a family, and we have the time to catch a favorite TV show like American Idol or Star Trek together.

In an ideal world, I'd be able to be on the go and participate in many of the activities that take Andy and Jakob away. But that's not a choice I get to make. My choice is between bitterness and acceptance; between maturing and refusing to grow. I don't want to get stuck in bitterness or anger or resentment. That means I have to die to my own desires a lot, and that's not fun, but I believe the temporary pain it causes builds character, and it makes me stronger. Suffering makes a clearer distinction between "needs" and "wants" in my life.

I'm thankful that when Jakob bursts in the front door, he wants to tell me about what he's experienced. He'll plop down in a chair and give me the highlights and lowlights of his experiences ... usually with just the right amount of exaggeration! He makes me laugh every day. I'm grateful to be his mom. And I'm so thankful to be Andy's wife—the one he wants to come home to at the end of his busy day. I can't *imagine* my life without him. Lately he's started taking a digital camera to events and snapping a bunch of photos, which I can look at on the laptop when he gets home. For years, he's been patiently taking the video camera and recording part of the concert or play that Jakob's been in. We all watch it together later, with its delayed action.

Sometimes, though, even the best of my coping skills falls short. I get totally frustrated, discouraged, and disheartened at all the things I want to do but can't. And sometimes, to my regret, I take it out on Andy ...

It's summer 2007, and the Tigers are having an awesome season. Andy and Jakob have driven in to Detroit to see a game at Comerica Park. It's gone late—into ten innings—and they pull into the driveway after midnight. Roxanne is waiting for them, having tried to pass the evening watching the Lifetime Network. She's agitated by pain and fatigue, but unable to sleep. She gives Jakob a quick hug, and he falls into bed, asleep in under sixty seconds.

Roxanne heads to bed, and after locking up the house, Andy joins her. She turns to him, "I had a hard time tonight."

"I'm sorry to hear that," Andy responds.

"Are you? Are you really? I didn't notice. You were too busy having fun."

"Hey, we agreed that I could go to the game with Jakob tonight. You said it was okay."

"I <u>know</u> I did, but it's just not fair! You and Jakob and everyone else on the planet get to go have fun. I <u>never</u> get to go do the fun things," Roxanne exclaims, the tension apparent in her voice.

"I don't know what to say. I tried to take you to a park yesterday for an hour, but your pain was too bad. It's so hard to find anything that works for us to do together."

"It's not just the baseball game tonight. It's that, and the trip to Cedar Point, and the bike ride you guys took last week. I just have to be okay with you guys getting to go places, but I have to stay home again, in pain. I <u>hate</u> that!"

"I hate that, too. But you always encourage me to take Jakob places," says Andy, throwing his hands out in frustration.

"I want Jakob to have these experiences, but I want to have them, too. I used to be the one who was athletic. I used to climb mountains and go skiing. Now you get to do all the active stuff. You don't deserve it any more than I do. And I have to watch all my friends go on their vacations and do all their sports and have more children, while I don't get any of that! They don't deserve it any more than I do, either!"

Roxanne is visibly torn between anger and sadness. She and Andy continue this type of heated conversation for the next five minutes. Finally, Roxanne asserts for the tenth time, "It's not fair!"

*"You're right: it isn't fair. I know you're upset, and you have a right to be angry, but don't be angry with me. Let's both be angry at the situation. And now isn't the best time to deal with this. I don't think we can solve this tonight." Andy turns toward Roxanne in bed, holding out his arms. She enters his embrace and begins crying into his shoulder. "Just let it out," he says. "You **have** to cry sometimes." Roxanne, knowing that Andy's giving her a safe place, lets herself go. The sobs shudder through her body, and finally sleep comes ...*

The next morning, Andy wakes up earlier than Roxanne, as usual. He's sitting at the table, sipping coffee and reading, when she walks into the room:

"Hi Andy, how's it going?"

"Oh, hey—you're up. Did you sleep well?" Andy's question is more than just social; insomnia is a very real part of Roxanne's life, especially after an emotional confrontation.

"Yeah, pretty well. I feel quite a bit calmer."

*"That's good. Things can look better
in the morning."*

*"I feel like I need to apologize to you for last night. I
really lost perspective," Roxanne offers.*

*"I know that things are harder for you in the evening,
after dealing with pain all day," Andy replies.*

*"Yeah, it's usually my worst time of the day, but it
doesn't excuse me for giving you a hard time. I'm
sorry about the things I said to you last night."*

"Come here. Let me give you a hug. It's okay."

*"Thanks, honey. This morning things don't look quite
so bleak. It's not that I'm happy that I can't go to ball
games and amusement parks with you guys, but I feel
like I can cope again."*

*"Maybe we could try to get you out of here for an
hour this morning. Just go somewhere—anywhere—
to give you a change of environment. Let's do what
we can for you."*

*"Okay, how about after breakfast? We could even just
bring a blanket and I could lie down in a park. I just
need a change."*

A short trip to a park is the best we can do, but it will never
satisfy me. I long for adventure. I used to climb for an entire

day in the Rockies or go white-water rafting for a weekend or go snorkeling on a coral reef in the ocean. Now I have to settle for lying on a picnic blanket in a local park.

That's when I think about Heaven. In Heaven there won't be any pain, tears, or limitations. I'll have a body that works in every way. There I'll be able to join Andy and Jakob in whatever they're doing! I might be able to lift Jakob up in the air and swing him around like I wanted to when he was a child. I'll be able to hike in the mountains for hours with Andy. The three of us can go golfing, or catch a baseball game. I'll be able to dance for joy.

CHAPTER NINE

Tweaking
Pain Management

Pain Patch: Transdermal Fentanyl

Whenit became obvious that even after the artificial disc surgery I was going to have to deal with severe daily pain, we decided to try increasing the pain medications. My cousin, Diane Graft, began talking to me about the idea of a "pain patch." Diane has a disability, too—in her case, very severe arthritis. We had developed a relationship of mutual support over several years, mostly through long distance phone calls. Like me, she had enjoyed a very active, normal childhood. Diane had become disabled in her late teens by severe juvenile rheumatoid arthritis. After completing a nursing degree in college, her disability prevented her from getting a job in active nursing. Instead, she worked at a desk job for several years at a large insurance company before going on long-term disability. Diane had been urging me to try the Fentanyl transdermal patch, which would allow another pain medication to enter my circulatory system through the skin. She had been using the Fentanyl patch with some success for over a year.

I went to a third pain clinic to be evaluated for this patch, since my current (second) pain clinic didn't prescribe it, preferring to focus on injections. My initial evaluation by an anesthesiologist there went well, and he gave me a prescription for the Fentanyl patch. In addition, he wanted me to be seen by a pain psychologist. Although I thought that interview went all right, the pain psychologist seemed surprised that I was lying down on a mat instead of sitting in a chair. He decided I was a "malingerer"—someone who feigned or exaggerated the symptoms of an illness or injury to gain something from it. Specifically, he believed I was faking my pain in order to get attention from my husband, and in order to make my husband take care of me! He came to this conclusion and presented it to the pain clinic team, recommending that I be put in an in-patient psychiatric ward, where I could be forced to function regardless of pain.

We were absolutely shocked at the lack of professionalism evident here. I brought in discogram films and postoperative reports, along with an MRI film documenting degenerative disc disease. Nevertheless, the pain clinic team ignored the physiological proof of tissue damage, choosing to listen to the pain psychologist instead. Incredibly, they made this decision in a vacuum, failing to consult with my referring neurologist, whom I'd seen for fourteen years! The pain psychologist also failed to consult my psychiatrist, who was treating me for depression but had never doubted that my pain was real. This pain clinic's judgment didn't fit my medical history. If I had been a "malingerer," why would I have tried so hard for so many years to get well?

Andy and I were truly outraged. How dare the pain psychologist pronounce judgment on me, when there was plenty of evidence of a real condition! He did not have to face my pain each day. If only I could transfer my pain to him for 24 hours, he'd quickly realize how very real and disabling it is. With no evidence at all, this psychologist prejudiced the rest of the team against me. My physical therapist, Pam, attended the pain clinic's team meeting. She said that the group of physicians and the pain psychologist were sitting around a conference table, acting insensitively and making light of the suffering of several different patients. Pam said the social worker present looked very uncomfortable with this but didn't speak up. Pam tried to introduce objective information about my condition, but they ignored her input. In the face of this completely unprofessional treatment, Pam conferred with Dr. Elkiss. Together they verified that I had real pathology, and that I was not malingering. They had each personally treated me, and they also had access to fourteen years of my medical records, so they were in a position to make a better judgment.

Being labeled a "malingerer" seemed particularly malicious. This was kicking somebody when they were already down—wounding a patient already burdened with suffering. And unfortunately, this is not a rare experience for people with chronic pain. To add insult to injury, they billed my insurance for several hundred dollars for the consultation. Not only did the pain clinic team fail to relieve any small part of my suffering, but they added a burden to my load. To actually help someone with long-term pain, the medical professional needs to start by believing the patient. In my second pain clinic I had been told of a statistic, that only one percent of patients with chronic pain are malingering—a very tiny minority. Assume pain is real for 99%.

So now I was on a low level of the pain patch but couldn't go back to the clinic which had prescribed it. The other clinic where I went for steroid injections didn't prescribe the Fentanyl patch. Fortunately for me, my primary care doctor, Dr. Arthur Tai, was willing to continue prescribing it for me. Because of FDA rules, he had to write a new prescription for me every month which couldn't be phoned in to the pharmacy but had to be picked up in person.

The patch releases twenty-five micrograms of Fentanyl per hour; each patch lasts seventy-two hours. This initial dose didn't relieve much of my pain, so my doctor increased it to fifty micrograms an hour. This dosage helped a little, but not nearly as much as I'd expected. I still had pain, and still needed to take Vicodin in addition to the patch. The side effects of nausea, constipation and itching were manageable, but the Fentanyl caused me severe insomnia every third day when I'd change the patch. I simply couldn't fall asleep until two or three in the morning. I was disappointed to discover that even with the patch, I still needed to lie down most of the time to manage my pain.

After a year on this medication, my primary care doctor tried switching me to an oral medication called Oxycontin, which is a slow-release opiate[*]. I took twenty milligrams of Oxycontin every twelve hours to treat my baseline pain, and I used Vicodin for breakthrough pain as needed. I had

---

[*] There are quick-release and extended-release opiates, or narcotics. The extended-release opiates are released into the blood stream over a twelve-hour period of time. They take time to build up in the blood stream. The quick-release opiates give faster pain relief, but they don't last as long.

less insomnia as a result. My experience has been that the Oxycontin dulls the baseline pain, but does not eliminate it, and I still must limit my activity to avoid severe pain. Sadly, I still need to lie down most of the time to manage my pain.

The only remaining pain control option is the implanted spinal cord pump, which delivers morphine directly into the fluid surrounding the spinal cord. I have not been evaluated for this, because I've been told I'm too young for it. I'm forty-four at the time of this writing, and my anesthesiologist recommended trying that option later in life due to its potentially serious complications.

To summarize, there are limits to how well my pain can be managed with medications, at least with the ones we've tried so far. And the side effects of opiates are significant. Besides the severe constipation, requiring laxatives and stool-softeners, there is some mental haziness and short-term memory loss. Jakob and Andy like to tease me about things that we've discussed that I've since forgotten, and there are times when I'm reading that I don't recall anything on the prior pages. That's a little startling for me. But I'm grateful to have these opiate medications, because they make the pain tolerable, if I also limit my activity to two hours out of bed, or so, a day. They make my life bearable.

Psychiatrist's Perspective

Dr. Anita Kumar-Gill has been my psychiatrist since 2004. She helped me cope with my despair after the artificial disc failed to relieve my pain. In contrast to the "pain psychologist" I'd seen, Dr. Kumar-Gill believed that my pain was real, and she tried to help me cope with the psychological effects of pain. She helped me to understand that long-term pain causes chemical changes in the brain, which affect mood, causing depression. She earned my trust by being consistently supportive and affirming. She persevered with medication changes until we found the right doses and combinations of two anti-depressant medications. After my depression was successfully treated, I still was in pain but could cope with it better. The pain wasn't able to distress my mood as much as before. Dr. Kumar-Gill graciously consented to writing her perspective for this book. The following are her words.

"When I first met Roxanne, she was depressed and in a state of desperation. Her story was very striking. It amazed me that her life had changed so dramatically in just a few short years. She was a horizontal woman, with a fire in her belly that would not go out. But, at the same time, she was on the verge of being a broken woman. There was an understanding and resolution that she may have to live the rest of her life in some degree of physical pain.

She never considered ending her life. She simply wanted to know what she could do to improve her life. I was concerned that she had never been treated for a Major Depressive Episode. I do not specialize in pain management, but the literature is clear that chronic pain results in physiologic changes which would make a person much more vulnerable to Depressive Disorders.

Roxanne was open to the idea of taking an anti-depressant medication and being in therapy. When I suggested any medication changes or any non-medication treatments, she always followed through.

Because of her commitment to wellness and her faith,

she went from depressed on the floor during only morning appointments, to sitting up in a chair with the assistance of a traction device at a half-hour lunch appointment. She drove herself the ten-minute trip to my office to see me. Roxanne treats herself with respect. And, while she defers to the judgment of specialists, she always knows what her limits are. She goes with her gut feeling.

Roxanne is a woman of resilience. We all are. We all have that same potential. Roxanne simply works harder than most of us to tap into that energy that allows us to thrive, despite the circumstances. She understands that her source of strength comes from within. Accessing that source may seem scary at first, and we should take our own paths and our own pace. But, Roxanne's story is evidence of the depth of the human spirit, and our innate ability to tolerate adversity. She is a reminder to us all that the limits that we experience are self-created. If we break down those bars, we are an unlimited possibility."

CHAPTER TEN

When It's All Said and Done

My story isn't over yet. We don't know if my pain will get worse or better in the future. All we know is that we've made the best choices we could, but that as of the present moment, I'm still disabled by pain. We don't know what plan God has for us, but we trust that He has one—and that, at least for the present, His plan includes suffering.

After eighteen years of this, I know some things. I know that suffering is harsh, hard, and even horrible at times. I know that it's especially demoralizing when it never ends! No one likes suffering, and few would normally choose it. A person can be completely overwhelmed at times by suffering, adrift at sea, buffeted by gale-force winds, facing seemingly insurmountable obstacles. At those times, it can seem like there are no limits to what suffering or loss can take away.

But the truth is, it can't take everything good away. Suffering can make you fear for the loss of who you are, and who you hope to become. It can change what you are able to do. But it can't take away your deepest identity as a human being and a child of God.

I was afraid that suffering carried a mandatory sentence of depression and anger. And there has been depression and anger. But that's not all there has been. 2 Corinthians 4:6–8 says it best:

> God made his light shine in our hearts, to give us the knowledge of the glory of God in the face of Christ. But we have this treasure in jars of clay (our human bodies), to show that this all-surpassing power is from God and not from us. We are hard pressed on every side, but not crushed; perplexed but not in despair; persecuted, but not abandoned; struck down, but not destroyed.

Suffering struck me down eighteen years ago. It stole my youth. It robbed me of my career. It put an end to my physical freedom. It sentenced me to a horizontal life, lived in pain. But it has NOT destroyed me. Suffering has not been able to take away all that's good in life.

There can still be *joy* in life, even in a life with suffering and deprivation. There are still moments of joy. I've found that my losses can lead me to bitterness and envy of others, but they can also bring me to greater levels of gratitude for simple things. Joy may spring out of the simplest moments in life—sharing a laugh with a friend; enjoying the presence of a child; petting a dog; holding a spouse's hand; eating a meal with others; receiving kindness from a stranger. I've learned to look for these moments and to notice them when they happen … appreciating them … living mindfully. I don't have the most accomplished life—at least the way people perceive accomplishment—or the life with the most perks, but at times I have joy. I also derive joy from knowing God's presence and His care for me. Psalm 16:11 comments on this joy:

> You have made known to me the path of life; You will fill me with joy in your presence, with eternal pleasure at your right hand.

There is *love*, as well, even in a life of suffering. If true love is the giving of self to another, suffering can enhance love, because it provides opportunities to give and to receive help in significant ways. Caregivers and friends can show love to the suffering person by serving them, encouraging them, including them in events and activities, and praying for them. The suffering person can show love to those around her or him by being sensitive to the suffering of others; having a greater understanding and empathy for loss; by being a good listener; and by praying for others. The suffering person can also show love by encouraging his or her caregivers to take a break or to do something they enjoy. Yes, there is still love. 1 Corinthians 13:13 says:

> And now these three remain: faith, hope, and love. But the greatest of these is love.

You can still have *hope* in the midst of suffering. I speak of a different hope than the primary hope for relief of suffering or hope for a cure. Those are good hopes, but not always possible to fulfill. When the suffering is not relieved, there can still be hope for the ability to cope with limitations and get on with living the best that one can ... adapting, accommodating, living with it. There is also the hope of growing up in one's faith, and of God's maturing a person through his or her pain. Romans 5:3–5 speaks to the mystery of suffering yielding *hope*, a very counterintuitive process:

> Let us rejoice in our sufferings, because we know that suffering produces perseverance; perseverance, character; and character, hope. And hope does not disappoint us because God has poured out his love into our hearts by the Holy Spirit, whom he has given us.

If you feel like you've lost hope altogether, that could be depression. As Dr. Kumar-Gill indicated earlier in this book, there is a strong physiological link between pain and depression. I'm under the care of a psychiatrist, and I take two anti-depressant medications. If you are feeling hopeless, please consider being screened for depression.

And finally, there is *meaning* in suffering. Pastor Koch used to say to me, "God doesn't waste suffering." He meant that if we do the hard work of suffering—and it is hard work— that God will bring something worthwhile and useful out of it. There is a mystery about *how* He uses it, and *what* He accomplishes through it, but there is no doubt that He *does use it* and *accomplishes things through it*.

Even as I write this, my beloved Pastor Koch is very ill with metastatic prostate cancer. As much as we pray for healing and long life for him, we also know by *faith* that God is accomplishing something even through this brutal battle with cancer. There are many New Testament references to

God refining us, pruning us, changing our hearts, changing our character, making us more Christ-like through suffering.

> For a little while you may have had to suffer grief and all kinds of trials. These have come so that your faith—of greater worth than gold, which perishes even though refined by fire—may be proved genuine and may result in praise, glory, and honor when Jesus Christ is revealed (1 Peter 1:6b–7).

I've had to surrender my life to God's care many times. I've told Him countless times that I don't understand why I have disabling pain, that I don't want to be so limited in what I can do, and that I would have chosen a very different life if it were up to me. But I've also asked God to use my life, humble as it is, for His purposes. I've asked Him to help me trust that He will give my suffering *meaning*. And He will give your suffering *meaning*, too. God is present and He will help you. He won't respond to your suffering in the same ways He responded to mine. God is not going to use a cookie-cutter approach; He's far more creative and personal than that. He will respond to your suffering in His ways and in His timing, in the ways which are best for you and others around you.

Be encouraged! There *is* purpose and meaning in your suffering. God *is* with you 100% of the way. There can still be joy, love, and hope during suffering. My hope and prayer for you is that you can keep going and keep facing your circumstances for another day. If you put your hope in God, He will strengthen you.

> The Lord gives strength to the weary, and increases the

power of the weak. Even youths grow tired and weary, and young men stumble and fall, but those who hope in the Lord will renew their strength. They will soar on wings like eagles; they will run and not grow weary, they will walk and not be faint (Isaiah 40:29–31).

Be empowered and uplifted by the lyrics of Darrell Evans' beautiful song, Trading My Sorrows:

I'm trading my sorrow
I'm trading my shame
I'm laying it down for the joy of the Lord

I'm trading my sickness
I'm trading my pain
I'm laying it down for the joy of the Lord

And we say yes Lord yes Lord yes yes Lord
Yes Lord yes Lord yes yes Lord
Yes Lord yes Lord yes yes Lord Amen

I'm pressed but not crushed persecuted not abandoned
Struck down but not destroyed
I'm blessed beyond the curse for his promise will endure
And his joy's gonna be my strength

Though the sorrow may last for the night
His joy comes with the morning

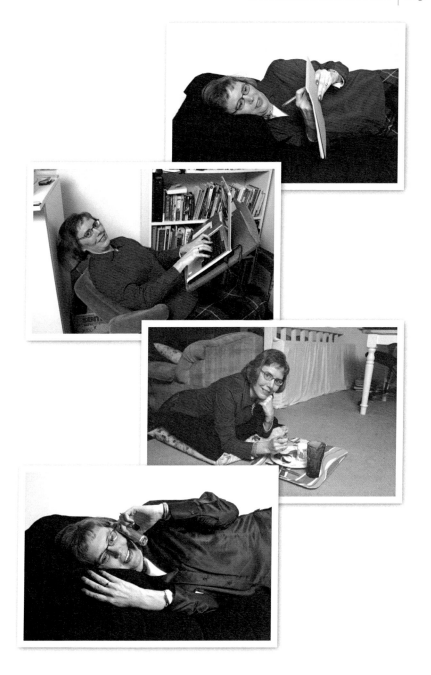

Roxanne at home.

EPILOGUE

Are You Hiding?
Seeking God's Touch

In early 2006, I experienced a prolonged pain flare that lasted several *months*. Suddenly, I had to cancel most of my usual activities, and I couldn't get back down to my usual level of pain. Spring turned to summer and the pain went on and on and on, day after day, week after week. We had to cancel our annual summer vacation to a log cabin in northern Michigan. I had a terrible time falling asleep at night because of the pain and because of my emotional distress from the pain. Taking pain medications dulled the pain, but made it even harder to sleep; taking sleeping pills let me sleep, but it was less effective sleep, and in the morning I felt weary and drugged. Once again desperation clung to me like a heavy cloak. Helplessness and hopelessness, like thick vines of groundcover, threatened to choke out the light. Once again, despair stalked me.

My mom asked me on the phone, "Did you see your doctor?" I had been keeping my usual appointments, but that didn't mean that anybody could help me. The limited efficacy of western medicine in my case had left me with few alternatives.

I sought God's help—not for the first time—but really having nowhere else to go. I prayed, not knowing how, when, where, or through whom He might choose to act. I knew I couldn't predict God. But I also knew that He would listen and respond in *some* way to my prayer. He had promised to respond in Psalm 50:15:

> Call on me in the day of trouble. I will deliver you and you will praise me.

Of course, God's idea of "delivering me" might not be the same way I wanted Him to respond ... but He would do *something* to help me.

There was just one problem: praying for healing simply wasn't good for me anymore.

I'd had many people pray with me for healing in the past, but I found those sessions to be immensely frustrating at this point. It was hard to ask God for the same thing—healing—over and over again. It's not as though if we prayed the right way, or used the right formula, God would give us a different answer. Praying for healing felt like *straining* toward a God who seemed distant and out of reach; I wanted to find a way to simply *receive* whatever He wanted to give me.

Reiki / Energy Medicine

The phone rang, and it was a therapist whom I'd contacted the year before, who now had an opening. Dr. Kumar-Gill, my psychiatrist, had found the therapist's name listed in a mental health directory under the category of "chronic illness." In addition to doing traditional psychotherapy, Dr. Copper[*] also did "energy work." I agreed to come for an initial appointment after she said that I could lie down on a massage table in her office.

My good friend Laurie drove me in my own van to the appointment. Every pothole in the street caused me agony. When I arrived at her office, Dr. Copper saw my distress, and she helped me to get settled on the massage table right away. Her kindness and her soft, soothing voice began calming me down. After a brief interview, she walked to the foot of the table where I was lying, facedown. She held both of my ankles and began "sensing" my energy flow. She seemed to be very intuitive, and she was able to tell me things about where energy was blocked or moving freely in my legs or back.

Dr. Copper's treatments of pressure, light touch, or even blowing were supposed to balance my "good" energy, "ground" my feet, and rid me of "bad" energy. While these techniques were unusual from my experience, she seemed to be quite skilled in them. I was fairly comfortable with all of it, until she began summoning various spirits into the room. She called the spirits individually by name, and she asked them to guide her energy work. Dr. Copper asked me whether I was in touch with the spirit world; I said, "With the Holy Spirit, I am." And she said, "So let it be." Shortly afterward, the treatment was over.

After getting home, Andy and I looked up Reiki on the Internet. It is a system designed to train practitioners to

---

[*] Name has been changed.

sense and to manipulate human energy fields. In theory, anyway, some people can perceive energy flowing through and around the human body. I ordered and read a book about the physics of this electromagnetic energy field which helped me to understand the concept.[1] With Reiki, the training process doesn't only involve learning to sense the physical electromagnetic field; there's also a spiritual element. During the training, Reiki healers are encouraged to invite "spirit guides" to assist them in their work. Some of the guides could be deceased Reiki masters. As a Christian, I didn't want to invite any other spirit into my life than the Holy Spirit; I wondered whether I might find a Christian Reiki practitioner.

We did an Internet search and found some Christian Reiki healers in California, but none in Michigan. After e-mailing a friend about my experience, she mentioned that there was a Christian "energy healer" at her workplace. I phoned him, and he was eager to come to my house to treat me. I arranged the appointment on a day when my sister would be visiting me, so that I wouldn't be home alone.

Jerry looked like an aging hippy. He had long hair in a ponytail, and he was thin and agile, moving easily. Jerry approached me where I was lying on my side on a daybed in our living room. He didn't touch my back or legs at all, but he started to make rapid movements in the air above me with his hands. He didn't try to sense the energy field. He seemed more interested in "pushing" the energy from his hand through my body to his other hand, and back again, without actually touching me.

---

[1] *Energy Medicine: The Scientific Basis* by James L. Oschman

Jerry told me stories of other people with whom he'd worked. He wanted me to "feel something" in my spine, and when that didn't happen, he became more insistent and "moved" the energy faster and faster. A couple of times, his hand actually hit me by accident—a rather startling and distressing experience. Although there was nothing here to make me uncomfortable spiritually, Jerry didn't seem to be very skilled in these techniques. I was growing increasingly uncomfortable with his approach, and the pressure to "feel something change." After an hour, I asked him to stop the treatment. I knew God wasn't leading me to this man; this treatment approach didn't give me any peace.

My understanding is that there is also a form of energy medicine called "therapeutic touch." I didn't explore this at all, so I can't comment about it.

Manual Lymph Drainage

Shortly after this, a woman from my church, who was a fellow Stephen Minister, offered to give me a free trial of something called "manual lymph drainage." I had never heard of this before but respected the fact that Carol was an occupational therapist. I decided to give it a try. Carol came to my house with a portable massage table. She explained that the lymph system returns fluid to the heart, but that sometimes lymph drainage gets blocked. It can be assisted by very light pressure in the direction of the heart. Carol thought there was at least a possibility that improving the return flow of my lymph might reduce my fluid retention and therefore my pain.

After having me lie down on the table, Carol proceeded to

apply light strokes with her fingers on my arms, trunk, and legs. The pressure was quite soft, about like the weight of a nickel. She played relaxing music during the treatment. Carol was very calm and quiet, and the treatment was very soothing. I realized how much I try to disconnect my head from my body because of the sensation of pain; Carol's treatment was reminding my brain that I have ankles and knees, forearms and shoulders which can feel pleasure, instead of merely a back that overwhelms me with pain. I set up several more treatment sessions with her.

Raindrop Therapy with Essential Oils

As my pain flare continued, though, Dr. Elkiss prescribed oral steroids in order to try to get the inflammation in my back under control. A deeper form of massage would complement the steroid treatment. So I asked another fellow Stephen Minister who had a massage business whether she could try working with me. Sherry worked with "essential oils" which had been extracted from plants, applying them systematically to the spine with massage techniques. The oils had health benefits completely aside from the massage strokes, which enhanced those effects. In addition, she used warm moist towels to heat my feet and my back while she was massaging other areas.

Sherry also played music during the treatment—spiritual songs about faith, trust, and surrender. These treatments went much deeper into the muscle than the manual lymph drainage, and my back responded more to them. It seemed that I'd finally found the right approach to receive God's touch. While both the prayer sessions for healing and the energy work had felt like *straining* toward God, this was simply *receiving* from Him. Sherry's touch represented God's touch to me. We set up regular treatment sessions. While this touch was reassuring to me, though, my pain flare continued.

Making Treatment Decisions

The intersection of faith and medicine is a complex place. On the one hand, some patients deal with this complexity by saying, "I'll work with any health care professional who seems to offer hope for improvement." On the other hand, there are those who say, "I'll only work with those health care providers who state that they have the same faith that I do." Both of these reactions seem too simplistic. I don't want to put limits on God's choice of healers for me, but I also don't want to engage in any practice which would contradict my understanding of the Holy Spirit. I've received wonderful care from health care practitioners and physicians of other faiths, who were genuinely helpful, and whose techniques and practices were still compatible with my faith.

Group Prayer for Direction

The other thing that Andy and I did in response to my pain flare and my resulting desperation was to invite a small group of friends over to our house. As a group, we would pray for God's leading and direction for me. To me, this was different from and far more comprehensive than praying only for physical healing, which had proven to be so frustrating in the past. About ten friends were able to make it, and they prayed that God would supply what I needed, physically, emotionally, and spiritually. I really felt like my burden of pain and suffering was shared during the group prayer time. It struck us that our friends cared as much as Andy and I did about my suffering and God's response to it. Pain is a burden which I have to carry alone so much of the time. It was extremely encouraging to know that others were helping me to carry the burden in prayer.

Neurosurgery Consultation

Although I didn't really want to see another doctor, by late summer my desperation for answers forced my hand.

I made an appointment with a surgeon about whom I'd heard for a couple of years. Dr. Tech Soo was chief of neurosurgery at Providence Hospital in Southfield, Michigan, about an hour from where we live. Dr. Soo had been working with the artificial disc in the U.S. since about 2003. I'd been waiting until he had a significant number of patient outcomes to potentially understand why some patients have so much pain after the artificial disc. Now seemed like a good time to schedule a consultation with him. Dr. Elkiss wrote a letter of introduction for me, and we went to see Dr. Soo. Maybe he could do a minimally invasive surgery just to remove the few rings of disc tissue left around my artificial disc. Maybe a microsurgery could help me.

Dr. Soo struck us as being energetic and a very quick decision-maker. However, he was also patient and had a surprisingly gentle voice and manner. Dr. Soo astonished us by saying that he strongly dislikes the artificial disc, and that a significant number of patients who receive one don't get better. He stunned us by proposing that he convert my artificial disc into a fusion! I told him that this was what we'd worked so hard to avoid, because it would lead to other fusions as the remaining discs were stressed more. "Exactly!" he replied, "your whole lumbar spine needs to be fused!" He told us that he'd need a new MRI and a discogram to know how many levels should be fused. I recoiled from the suggestion of the discogram, but he convinced me that it was a necessary test in order to proceed toward a surgery that might relieve some of my pain. Then he looked me straight in the eye and said, "You've been through the wringer, you poor thing. I'm so sorry that you've had to suffer for so many years with this. I know what's wrong, and I know how to help you. This surgery is not technically difficult for me."

Those were such compelling words, at a time when Andy and I had nearly given up ever hearing them from anyone again. We desperately wanted to believe him. Somehow, during the brief office visit we had with Dr. Soo, he earned our trust. We were surprised by his compassion. Although Andy and I found a sense of hope in his optimism, I was very reluctant to undergo another discogram, because it is such an excruciating test. But undergo it I did. My fourth discogram showed disc degeneration at two levels: the level of the artificial disc, and the level below it. Dr. Soo proposed a two-level fusion surgery, from L2 to L4, with L4 through S1 already having been fused. After the surgery, all of my lower back would be fused, except for the highest level, L1/L2. I wouldn't ever be able to bend my back forward, backward, or sideways again.

Andy and I discussed Dr. Soo's recommendations. We weren't sure whether or not Dr. Soo's ideas would prove to be right for me, but we decided that God was leading us in this direction. Andy and I both had peace about this path, this bend in the maze of suffering. And following God's leading, whether in the presence or absence of success, was what we'd done for sixteen years.

Surgery

I underwent this major surgery—my fourth spine surgery—in October 2006. It was my most invasive and traumatic surgery to date—nothing like a microsurgery! Dr. Soo stabilized the fusions with eight three-inch screws from the back to the front of my spine, two through each vertebral body, from L2 to L5. The screws were connected posteriorly by a series of metal struts. When I saw the post-op X-rays for the first time, I nearly fainted. My post-operative pain was uncontrollable for the first five days that I was an inpatient. They gave me so much morphine that my respiration rate and blood pressure dipped dangerously low. Yet the pain remained intense.

The day I was discharged, Andy drove me home in our van, and I cringed when we hit rough spots on the highway. When you're flying down the interstate at seventy miles an hour, it's hard to avoid all the potholes. By the time we reached our driveway, tears were streaming down my cheeks. I slowly made my way from the van to our front door, crying as I took each step with a walker.

This was my most extensive surgery yet, and the recovery was agonizingly slow and painful. My wonderful sister Barb flew up from Atlanta to stay with me so that Andy could return to work. I had to use a walker just to move around the house. I couldn't even put socks on, because there was no mobility in my spine, so I couldn't bend forward to reach my feet. My neighbor Betty offered to drive me to the mall where I pushed a rolling walker at a snail's pace, 100-200 feet, three mornings a week. I lived in sweat pants because I couldn't stand to wear anything close-fitting around my waist. My incision was ten inches long!

We tried to look for early signs as to whether there would be any gains from the surgery. Initially, I was able to eat one meal per day sitting up at the table for twenty minutes. We were encouraged by that. If only that would last, the surgical pain would have been worth it. I was walking a little further and faster each week, and I retired my walker. I resumed water therapy at the pool.

Unfortunately, though, as I gradually weaned off the very strong post-op pain medications, it became obvious that my pre-surgical pain levels were unchanged. At my six-month post-op visit with Dr. Soo, he took new X-rays. The fusions had been successful, in that the bone cells had grown between my vertebrae. The fusions had solidified. But my pain was no better. Dr. Soo's face looked sober as he asked me, "How many spine surgeries have you had?" "Four," I answered. He shook his head sadly and commented, "There are some people that we just can't help." What a contrast from his statement six months earlier: "I know what's wrong, and I can help you."

We drove home from the six-month appointment stunned, having been discharged from Dr. Soo's care. How could my pain still be so vicious and disabling? How could this promised and hoped-for improvement elude us once again? Why was it that other people get pain relief after surgery but I never do?

I'd already been through this enormous "let-down" phase once, after the 2003 surgery, and I saw it coming at me again.

Dr. Kumar-Gill and I scanned a list of local psychologists, and found the name "Dr. Dorella Bond" under the heading "Pastoral Care," because I knew that accepting another devastating disappointment was going to involve my faith.

We simply don't have complete answers for the "why"s. We will grieve this outcome once again. We will strive yet again for acceptance of our circumstances. We have the comfort of knowing we tried everything possible to help me.

Dr. Bond's greatest gift to me has been her encouragement to go places more often while lying down. I've been self-conscious and hesitant to do this, but she has been persuasive in reassuring me that my limitations are what they are, and that I need not be self-conscious about being a "horizontal woman" in public settings. Dr. Bond has repeatedly asserted that I haven't done anything wrong, but society has been in the wrong for not being willing to accept or accommodate someone who is different from the norm, even the norm for disability. And so my narrow life has opened just a little bit wider. So with her encouragement, I am getting out more on my cot: to a play in a small theatre that was willing to accommodate me, to a fireworks show, and to a class at the library. And that's a type of healing of its own.

~ ⌖ ~

Appendix A: Thoughts for Caregivers

It may sound like a cliché, but I experience God's love by experiencing the love of His people: receiving cards, meals, visits, or having someone give me a ride is enormously helpful and encouraging. These people represent Jesus to me. When you as a caregiver choose to do something for the suffering person, you become Jesus to them.

At the same time, I don't want to be on the receiving end and never have anything to contribute. Help the person find things they can do, and affirm their contribution, however large or small. Keep in mind that there are contributions which don't involve physical work: active listening, being an encourager, praying, writing, tutoring, helping a child with reading, but which still make a difference.

Be flexible. Because a person with pain will have good days and bad days, be ready to alter plans. Go ahead and do some things the person with limitations can't do, but also choose times to simply be with that person. Even if it means giving up activities you enjoy, you're doing it for the sake of the relationship. If you follow these suggestions, it will be better for everyone's mental health.

Listen. The suffering person needs to be heard. Try to put yourself in her or his shoes. Enter into that world for a few minutes. Then reflect back what you've heard, to be sure you understand. Accept her or his feelings. Point out anything you see the suffering person doing well, in terms of coping with the suffering. Try to encourage with a word of praise.

You don't have to be the only caregiver. Consider your role as being part of a team which may include family members, friends, a Stephen Minister, pastor, a psychologist or therapist, psychiatrist, or support group. Don't try to be a "Lone Ranger" caregiver... you need the other team members to do their part, too.

Appendix B: Thoughts for Sufferers

If suffering forces a radical shift in your lifestyle, give yourself time to grieve your losses. Cry, write in a journal, talk with a trusted confidant and to God, process your feelings of sadness or anger for as long as it takes. Be encouraged, though—time helps you adjust to the new lifestyle, and it does get easier. You may get to a point where you stop comparing your life with pain to your former life without it. Instead, you are comparing recent years with the pain to early years with the pain. You can feel good about your growing ability to cope, and the lessons you've learned about adapting. I'm doing a better job managing with the problem now than I was able to do when it first started.

Don't use one-upmanship. Don't compare suffering or minimize the suffering of others. Playing the comparison game is destructive and misses the whole point of growing in your ability to empathize with others who are in pain.

In relationships with friends and family, compromise. Choose times to free them up to do things you can't do without making them feel guilty. At other times, ask them to do something with you, even if it is more limited than they prefer, for the sake of your relationship. Recently, I attended a family reunion where the weather was so hot that no one wanted to go anywhere, and instead "hung out" at my parents' home for four days. No one left to do things I couldn't do. It was my favorite reunion ever! At other reunions, however, I had to let people come and go. I strove to content myself with spending time with them sporadically.

Try not to be self-conscious or ashamed if you look different from the norm. Hold your head high, look other people in the eye, and tell yourself you're doing a good job. It takes **courage** to be different ... affirm yourself for having that courage.

If people approach you with the latest medical cure, they may imply that you have nothing to lose by trying it. Thank them for their concern, but correct this misinformation by saying, "Actually, I do have to weigh my choices carefully. I only have so much time, money, and emotional resources, so I can't try everything." If you decide to try a new treatment, change only one thing at a time so you can assess its effect.

Practice assertiveness in your relationships ... not aggressiveness, but assertiveness. Tell people what you need. Calmly and politely repeat your request until someone listens. You can't afford to play games with people, pretending everything is all right when it isn't. Your relationships will work best if you learn to "speak the truth with love."[1]

Find more avenues of support than your closest family member or friend, and occasionally share your feelings with this second line of support. Living with pain affects you emotionally and spiritually so you need encouragement and empathy, but you don't want to burn out your support system. Try not to make the people closest to you a regular target for your anger or depression. Those closest to you also need your love, your time, and your empathy. They need you to be in a relationship with them that includes—but is not limited to—suffering.

We all like to make plans, but sometimes pain forces us to cancel those plans. If you have to "pull the plug" on plans to do

[1] *Speaking the Truth in Love: How to be an Assertive Christian*, by Ruth N. Koch and Kenneth C. Haugk Ph.D.; cf. Paul's letter in the New Testament.

something at the last minute, consider your options. Can you reschedule? Modify an activity? If children are involved, they can be quite disappointed at last-minute changes. Can you offer them a compromise? E.g., if we have to cancel a family outing because of my pain, we try to give Jakob something he'd like, such as a trip to Coldstone Creamery, rather than tell him to "buck up" and deal with the disappointment.

Celebrate small victories. Anything that connects you to people, anything which helps you take a small step toward a goal or allows you to make a contribution, is a victory.

Appendix C: Point System

If you want to try making a point system, it will need to be individualized for you and your situation. You may have a back that can sit for hours but only stand for a few minutes. You may have a completely different condition which limits you, like multiple sclerosis, cerebral palsy, or a spinal cord injury. Or you may have forty possible points of function, where I have only ten. If that's the case, you may want to define one point as a whole hour of some activity, and then limit yourself to ten.

Figure out which activities take a toll on you, and assign them points as I've done. Then write them down in a "points journal" each day, and try to learn what effect individual activities have on your pain. Be patient: this may take several weeks or even months, because your activity levels are not the only factor affecting your pain. For example, the weather with its barometric pressure changes might affect your pain. Whether you've slept well or poorly can make a difference. Emotional stress can worsen pain, as your muscles tighten up and your body processes stress-related chemicals. For women, menstrual cycles can affect pain levels. Gradually, though, over time, you'll be able to separate these factors out. Notice patterns of cause and effect.

Here's a sample of my point system:

Point System—2007

One Point Items:

- Clean up kitchen: simple

- Walk for five minutes
- Sit for ten minutes
- Stand still for twenty minutes
- Stand and move around for thirty minutes
- Organize a room for fifteen minutes
- Drive for ten minutes
- Be driven in the passenger seat for thirty minutes
- Be driven on the mattress in the back of the van for forty-five minutes
- Work for thirty minutes leaning forward on the step
- Computer work for thirty minutes leaning backward in a chair
- Light shopping thirty minutes (light lifting - one pound) not incl. drive time
- Fold dry clothes
- Having a visitor (one-and-a-half-hours)
- Stabilization exercises

Two Point Items:

- Clean up kitchen: complex
- Walk for ten minutes
- Basic physician appointment
- Physical therapy appointment in home
- Play a family game lying down
- Sit twenty minutes (rarely possible)
- Go to church (be driven, use daybed)
- Try on clothes: tops—fifteen minutes
- Organize Andy's wardrobe—fifteen minutes
- Host several friends—two hours

Three Point Items:

- Walk fifteen minutes
- Extended physician appointment
- Physical therapy appointment at clinic
- Visit a friend's house—lying on cot
- Small group meetings

Notes:

- Points need to be combined: e.g., a doctor visit may be two points, but it costs three points by the time you add in the driving.

- There are trade-offs and choices: I can choose to scrapbook photo albums while sitting for ten minutes; while standing for twenty minutes; or while leaning forward over a step for thirty minutes.

- Anything after 1 PM costs an extra point; anything done after 5 PM costs two extra points.

- I don't need to record all these extra charges, but simply keep them in mind; it's easiest on my back to do things early in the day.

Appendix D: Resources

Beers, V. Gilbert *Finding Purpose in Your Pain*

Berger, Suzanne E. *Horizontal Woman*

Brandt, Paul and Yancey, Philip *Fearfully and Wonderfully Made*

Christenson, Larry *Ride the River*

Copen, Lisa *Mosaic Moments: Devotions for the Chronically Ill*

Dobson, James *When God Doesn't Make Sense*

Haugk, Kenneth *Distinctively Christian Caregiving*

Haugk, Kenneth *Don't Sing Songs to a Heavy Heart: How to Relate to Those Who Are Suffering*

Koch, Ruth N. and Haugk, Kenneth C. *Speaking the Truth in Love: How to Be An Assertive Christian*

Kreeft, Peter *Making Sense Out of Suffering*

Lewis, C.S. *The Problem of Pain*

MacNutt, Francis *Healing*

Miller, Ruth L.S. *Lessons from the Washing Machine: Living with Reflex Sympathetic Dystrophy*

Nielsen, Patricia D. *Living With It Daily: Meditations for People with Chronic Pain*

Partow, Donna *This Isn't the Life I Signed Up For*

Spitzer, Robert J. *Healing the Culture*

Tada, Joni Eareckson and Estes, Rev. Steve *When God Weeps* (Especially Appendix B: Scriptures on God's Purpose in Our Sufferings, pp. 232–240)

Tada, Joni Eareckson *Heaven: Your Real Home*

Veith, Edward Gene *The Spirituality of the Cross*

Yancey, Phillip and Brandt, Paul *Pain: The Gift Nobody Wants*

Yancey, Phillip *Where's God When It Hurts?*

Zimmerman, Julie *Chronic Back Pain: Moving On*

Other Resources

Websites: Christian

Rest Ministries: restministries.org
Joni & Friends Disability Organization: joniandfriends.org

Websites: Other

American Chronic Pain Association: theacpa.org
Chronic Pain Support Groups: chronicpainsupport.org
Medicine Net: medicinenet.com/chronic_pain
National Chronic Pain Society: chronicpain.org
Society for Neuroscience: sfn.org
U. S. Food and Drug Administration: fda.gov

Index

A

Acupuncture 61, 75, 77
Adaptations 10, 78, 81, 90, 139,
142
Anesthesia 95, 120
Anger 19, 32, 92, 177, 185, 187,
203, 204, 207, 220, 243,
244
Artificial disc 121, 122, 123,
124, 131, 133, 134, 140,
144, 165, 166, 168, 172,
175, 176, 178, 211, 215,
234, 235

B

Biofeedback 61
British 141, 142, 150, 157, 159,
160, 167

C

Caregiver 10, 85, 90, 241, 242
Caregivers 11, 221, 241
Chronic pain 44, 45, 46, 69, 77,
86, 96, 138, 139, 213,
214, 216, 257
Courage i, 5, 113, 114, 137, 143,
144, 145, 158, 166, 182,
192, 244
CT 18, 43, 132, 140

D

Depression 5, 32, 91, 212, 216,
220, 222, 244
Despair 39, 177, 215, 220, 227
Disability 4, 9, 10, 11, 15, 18,
28, 45, 46, 55, 65, 68, 78,
81, 86, 87, 90, 60, 114, 89,
90, 91, 94, 98, 102, 104,
105, 112, 119, 121, 125,
130, 139, 141, 142, 147,
154, 177, 179, 180, 181,
183, 188, 191, 192, 193,
200, 203, 204, 238, 252
Disc i, 1, 14, 20, 21, 22, 23, 39,
44, 54, 56, 58, 59, 83, 91,
109, 113, 119, 120, 121,
122, 123, 124, 131, 132,
133, 134, 140, 144, 145,
163, 164, 165, 166, 168,
172, 175, 176, 178, 211,
212, 215, 234, 235
Discogram 55, 56, 120, 132,
140, 212, 235

E

EMG 18
England 10, 123, 131, 132, 140,
141, 142, 144, 150, 156,
157, 158, 160, 161, 162,
164, 165, 167, 168, 169,
172, 175, 178, 180, 186,
192
English 153, 158
Exercise 1, 63, 64, 68, 93, 113,
148, 149, 188, 62

F

Faith i, 5, 6, 13, 29, 30, 49, 51,
52, 94, 99, 113, 116, 144,
145, 185, 186, 187, 188,
194, 216, 221, 222, 223,
232, 233, 237

About the Author

ROXANNE M. SMITH is a
physical therapist whose life
changed suddenly at age twenty-
seven, when she became disabled
by severe pain. She has lived as a
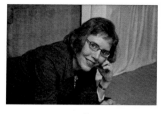
"horizontal woman," spending twenty or more hours a day
lying down, for eighteen years at this writing. She has endured
four major spine surgeries to date. Roxanne was trained
and works as a Stephen Minister, and she has served in her
congregation's parish health program. She has developed a
ministry to people with chronic pain or disabilities. She has
written articles for newsletters, magazines, and anthologies.
Roxanne and her family live in Michigan.

Visit her website at: www.RoxanneSmith.org

To order additional copies of *Struck Down but Not Destroyed* or to find out about other books by Roxanne M. Smith or Zoë Life Publishing please visit our website www.zoelifepub.com.

A bulk discount is available when 12 or more books are purchased at one time for your ministry, store, office or organization.

Zoë Life Publishing

P.O. Box 871066

Canton, MI 48187

(877) 841-3400

outreach@zoelifepub.com